5-Minute Strength Training Workouts for Seniors Over 60

3 Books In 1

150+ Power-Packed Exercises to Restore Flexibility, Improve Posture, Build Balance and Prevent Falls | Step-by-Step Instruction & Illustrations

Baz Thompson

Core Exercises for Seniors

Build Strength and Improve Stability for Active Aging After 60

Baz Thompson

Contents

Balance Exercises for Seniors

Before You Start Reading

What's in it for me?

- 101 highly effective strength training exercises that can help you reach the highest point of your fitness performance
- Foundational exercises to improve posture and increase range of motion in your arms, shoulders, chest, and back
- Stretches to help you gain flexibility and find deep relaxation
- Workout Logbook to help you keep track of your accomplishments and progress. Log your progress to give you the edge you need to accomplish your goals.

OR SCAN THE QR CODE

INTRODUCTION

You are looking forward to growing older with vitality and grace. But maybe you aren't sure how to achieve that. The good news is that you are reading this book. That means that you are hungry for information and willing to learn! In this instructional and practical guide, you will learn all about one of the pillars of active aging: a strong core.

Along with balance, strength, and flexibility, core strength is something you don't want to grow older lacking. You may currently have a weak or compromised abdominal and back muscle because of injury or surgery. On the other hand, perhaps you have a moderately strong core and want to take preventative measures to keep that strength as you age. Regardless of where you are physically, you can benefit from strengthening your core through exercise. We will travel this road together, learning about our bodies, how to keep them strong, and what simple choices we can make to ensure that we age well.

What are some everyday tasks that our core helps us to achieve? Just about everything!

- Sitting in a chair
- Getting up from the floor, bed, or chair
- Turning to look behind you
- Picking up items, bags, or packages
- Bending over to tie your shoes
- Getting dressed
- Taking a bath or shower
- Reaching for items overhead
- Vacuuming, mopping, sweeping
- Hammering, cutting, turning a screwdriver
- Physical activities like swimming, biking, bowling, golfing, tennis, rowing, running, walking

Our core must remain strong to retain our capacity to do these basic tasks. If not, we may require the assistance of others and lose our ability to live and work independently.

All our muscles, including those in our core, gradually lose mass and strength as we get older. While some of this may be due to injuries, surgeries, or illnesses, we often lose muscle strength because of inactivity. As a result, we fail or forget to train and work the muscles we need to stay strong. The good news? With regular exercise, we can regain and maintain strength in our muscles, particularly our core muscles.

ABOUT THIS BOOK

We will cover a lot of ground in this book, but it is all practical and easy-t0-understand information. The first part of the book helps develop a foundational understanding of our bodies, particularly our core. The second part of the book comprises the actual core exercises, broken down by the position in which they are done. And the last part of the book includes the practical application.

- ○ In Chapter 1, we will see a brief overview of aging and how we can slow the loss of muscle mass. Also covered is an outline of the core muscles and how a strong core benefits our daily living. Finally, there is a quick core strength quiz to help you assess your condition.

- ○ Chapter 2 goes into how we can develop core strength. No special equipment is needed! Common mistakes are revealed and helpful tips for making the most of your exercise time.

- ○ Mat core exercises are the focus in Chapter 3. Do you think this chapter is all about sit-ups? Think again! Featured are twelve of the best core exercises you can do while lying down. Spoiler alert: no sit-ups or crunches are involved.

- ○ In Chapter 4, seated core exercises are the focus. Many people are surprised to learn how safe, low-impact, and effective seated exercises can be for people of any age. Twelve powerful core exercises are highlighted and can all be done in a chair.

- ○ Chapter 5 concentrates on standing core exercises and training your core muscles while standing gives you the element of surprise. It mixes up your training routine and allows muscles to be worked differently. Spotlighted are twelve standing core strengtheners.

- ○ If you have a spouse, partner, or workout buddy, you will enjoy Chapter 6. This section is devoted to core exercises that you can do with a partner. These eight exercises are challenging and fun.

- ○ Chapter 7 calls attention to warm-up exercises and cool down stretches. These can be easy to overlook or forget, but it's essential to take a few minutes before exercising to prime our bodies and after exercising to let them unwind.

- ○ Chapter 8 outlines one of the primary ways to exercise and work our core: walking! There is a brief description of the best walking tips, along with six of the best ways to incorporate core exercises into your daily walk.

- ○ The action plan is revealed in Chapter 9. There are three weeks of workout routines for you to choose from or work through in this chapter. Each week features six days of core exercises.

HOW TO USE THIS BOOK

Not only will you learn about your core and the benefits of a strong core, but you will also find fifty core exercises that you can start doing today. In addition, there are ten exercises to help you get warmed up and cooled down. This book can be used as a guidebook and reference that you can turn back to again and again as you learn to strengthen your core.

Each exercise in this book will feature the following:

- name of the exercise
- time needed per rep
- total time to complete the exercise
- easy step-by-step instructions
- a variation of the exercise or a way to level up and make the exercise more challenging
- safety tips and things to watch out for to avoid injury

Illustrations accompanying each exercise will show you the correct positioning of your body, head, hands, and feet.

You can use this book in various ways, depending on your interests, abilities, and needs. One way is to work through each exercise, one-by-one, chapter-by-chapter systematically. Another way is to make up your exercise routine, picking the exercises you want to do each day. Or, to make life easy, you can take advantage of the weekly schedules at the end of the book and follow these. Find a system that you can stick to and that works for you. A stronger core awaits you and can be achieved with a bit of effort!

Getting older is unavoidable. But losing muscle mass and strength in our bodies does not have to go along with that. Becoming educated about how our bodies function, learning how we can slow down muscle loss, deciding to take steps to better our health, and putting in the effort to follow through with action will determine whether we age well or age. In writing this book, one of my goals is to encourage you on your health and well-being journey. So, we can all enjoy an active and strong second half of our lives. I hope that you will find this book a helpful resource as you strengthen your core and build your stability.

Please consult with your doctor before starting on any new exercise or activity.

My hope and desire is that you will find this book to be a valuable resource as you struggle to regain and maintain good balance in order to avoid falls and improve your general health. Are you all set? Let's get your fitness education and training started!

The Power of Your Core

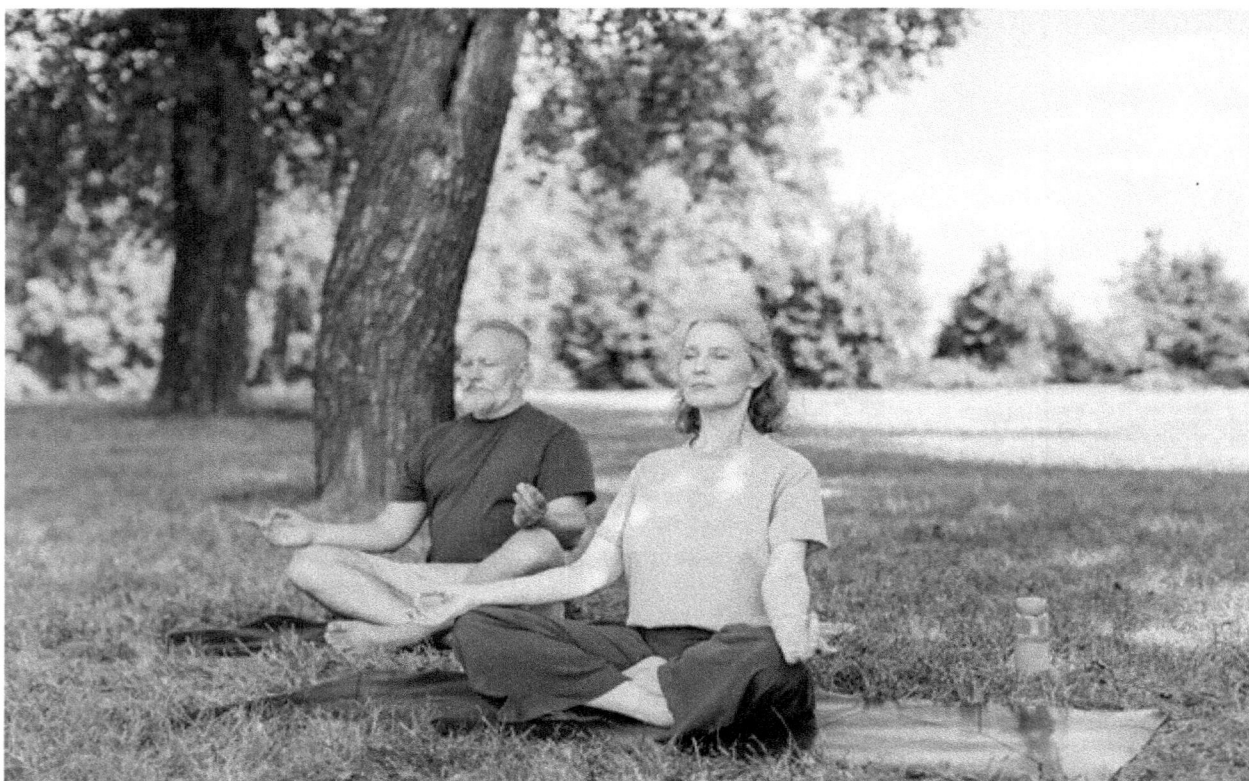

Age is inevitable. Aging isn't. —Marv Levy

Strong core muscles are a crucial part of our health and well-being. But they are also important to keep us physically mobile and stable. Our stability ensures that we can do certain tasks without the assistance of others as we get older. This helps us to stay independent for a longer period of time. In this chapter, we will take a brief look at what happens to our bodies as we progress in years. Next, we will examine what muscles make up our core muscles. We will define the benefits of having a strong core. Finally, there is a short quiz that can help determine whether our core is strong or lacking.

OUR BODIES AND AGING

Getting older is a natural part of life. However, once we hit 60 years of age, we may be labeled as old. This was perhaps true in the past centuries when life spans were shorter and living to age 60 was unusual. But presently, older adults live full and active lives well into their eighth and ninth decades of life. The older population is divided into three subcategories:

- Young-Old (ages 65 to 74)
- Middle-Old (ages 75 to 84)
- Old-Old (ages 85 and older)

The physical abilities and strengths of someone who is 65 years old can vary greatly from someone who is 85 years old, depending on their mental acuity, fitness level, and overall health. Besides age, a variety of factors can contribute to this difference, including foods eaten, exercise, weight, enriching activities, and adequate sleep.

Chronological age is something we cannot control, but biological age is reflected by the choices we make. For example, a 72-year-old may have battled breast cancer. This person chooses to consume a diet consisting of lean proteins, fresh fruits, and fresh vegetables. They can still play golf twice a week, practice stretching exercises daily, and complete jigsaw puzzles regularly. Another 72-year-old may suffer from a little arthritis in the hands and not have any other major health issues but chooses to eat a diet high in processed foods, salt, and sugar. They have constant brain fog, don't exercise, and spend most of their day sitting inside watching television. These two 72-year-olds are the same age chronologically, but biologically they are aging at different rates.

The human body is composed of many different types of cells. Some are short-lived and constantly being replaced, like skin cells. Others are long-lived but are never replaced, like brain cells. Muscle cells are self-renewing. As we age, however, we lose muscle mass and strength, contributing to increased frailty and instability. Slowing down the loss of muscle can be achieved with just a few changes in our lifestyle. A 2018 study by McCormick and Vasilaki recommended paying attention to the following factors to help maintain muscle mass and strength:

- Increased protein intake. Nearly 40% of people over 50 years old do not consume adequate amounts of protein.

- Aerobic exercise. Walking, running, cycling, and swimming stimulate the heart and blood flow to muscles while increasing lung capacity.

- Resistance training. Lifting weights, bodyweight exercise, and resistance bands stimulate skeletal muscles to grow and become stronger.

- Other physical activities. Stretching, yoga, and core exercises bring flexibility and strength to muscles.

Choosing to make changes to our daily life can help slow the loss of muscle strength and core stability as we grow older.

WHAT IS YOUR CORE

It is common to think that your core is just your abdominal muscles. Your abs are definitely part of your core, but there are nearly 35 muscles that make up this "torso girdle" that supports the body.

The main core muscles include:

- Rectus abdominis. This is what most people think of as "6 pack muscles" at the front of your abdomen. These muscles run from under your rib cage to your pubic bone.
- Obliques. Internal and external oblique muscles are on the sides of your torso. These muscles help you twist and turn your body.
- Transverse abdominis. This muscle holds your pelvis and internal organs in place.
- Erector spinae. These muscles are in your back along the spine and help you stand erect.
- Gluteus maximus. Located in your buttocks, these muscles assist you in lifting your legs, walking, and climbing stairs.

This brief overview gives you an idea of what some of these muscles do in supporting the body. There are several other core muscles not mentioned here that also play an important role.

THE RISK FACTORS OF A WEAK CORE

Lisa was a mother and grandmother that enjoyed being around her family. One of her favorite things to do with her granddaughters was to teach them how to plant flowers and vegetables in the garden. She had learned how to garden from her grandmother and loved working the earth to yield beautiful blooms and produce. At one time, Lisa was an avid dancer, but because of occasional arthritis in her knees, she did not dance as much anymore. In fact, she shied away from exercise of any kind because she did not enjoy the repetitive movements of most exercise routines. She preferred the freer expression of dance. One weekend, Lisa was lifting a heavy bag of potting soil from the trunk of her car and lost her balance. She fell in her driveway. Her arm braced her as she fell, but it was broken in two places as a result of landing on the concrete. Lisa spent the next few months recuperating from a broken arm, unable to garden with her granddaughters.

In the United States, one out of four older adults falls annually. Twenty-six million falls were reported in 2018, and that number increases from year to year. Falls are the leading cause of injury in adults over the age of 65 and are blamed for millions of injuries. What is causing older adults to fall? There are a variety of reasons, including impaired eyesight, slower reflexes, medications that cause dizziness, tripping hazards, and low blood pressure. Another primary reason for falls is the loss of balance and stability resulting from a weak core. The strength and flexibility of our back, abdominal, and buttock muscles determine our ability to react and adjust to changes in certain situations.

Some risks of having a core that cannot support you adequately include:

- Increased pain. Weak core muscles cause your pelvis to tilt and other muscles to pull on your spine, resulting in lower back and neck pain.
- Poor posture. Shoulders that hunch forward, a neck that cranes out, and a spine that is not in alignment are all indicators of a weak core.
- Imbalance and instability. Loss of balance results from your muscles being unable to keep you supported and stable as you twist, turn, reach, and lift. These imbalances can lead to falls.
- Fatigue. Loss of breath, inability to lift or carry items and overall sense of weakness are indicators of weak core muscles.

Loss of strength and stamina in your core muscles can infringe on your abilities and overall well-being.

THE BENEFITS OF STRENGTHENING YOUR CORE

Debbie and Tom loved camping. They both enjoyed the outdoors and had gone camping since they first started dating in the 1970s. As they raised their children, they did plenty of tent camping and taught their kids how to set up tents, haul water, and make a campfire. Once Tom turned 65, they decided to splurge and buy an RV so they could travel and camp all along the coastline. Debbie and Tom were both active in their local paddleball club and played several times a week. Even though they were in their early 70s, they didn't have any trouble driving their RV, maneuvering up and down the vehicle stairs, or reaching up to secure the awnings when they packed up, thanks to their legs and core muscles being strong. It is easy to take our core muscles for granted. But someone with impaired abdominal and back muscles would have had a difficult time doing some of the things in the above scenario. Going up and down narrow stairs, lifting and lowering awnings, and even handling a larger recreational vehicle can be tiring and possibly hazardous for someone who lacks core strength.

Is having a strong core the same as having well-defined six-pack abs? Not exactly. Having a strong core is more than just a nice physical appearance. Training and building your core muscles results in real-life benefits that affect your overall quality of life. Let's look at some of the benefits of having a well-toned core.

- Reduced Pain. Other areas of your body, such as the lower back and neck, don't have to compensate when the muscles that support your midsection and back are toned and strong.

- Good Posture. The muscles in your back and on the sides of your body, as well as the inner core muscles that attach to your spine, help you stay erect and upright.

- Better Balance and Stability. Having torso muscles that are sturdy helps provide a solid foundation for keeping you stable and staying on balance.

- Inner Organ Protection. The organs inside our midsection, like the stomach, liver, and kidneys, are protected by the muscles of our core. Having a muscular shield to deflect any potential damage helps keep them safe from injury.

A strong core is good for our physical bodies, but it's also central to things going smoothly in our everyday lives. Many tasks and functions are more difficult when our core muscles are not as strong as they could be. Some common everyday tasks that are helped by a strong core include:

- Driving a car
- Putting away groceries
- Exercising
- Holding a grandbaby
- Running errands
- Playing with grandkids
- Walking your dog
- Dancing with your partner

These everyday activities can be hindered or more difficult if your core muscles are not strong and flexible. A strong core contributes to maintaining a healthy and active lifestyle as you grow older. It also helps you to stay stronger longer. We all want to live independently without needing assistance.

TEST YOUR CORE

How strong is your core? You can discern if your core could benefit from strengthening by taking the quiz below. Be honest in your answers. No one is judging you or your abilities.

CORE STRENGTH QUIZ

The answer choices are: Yes or No.

1. From a seated position on the floor or a chair, can you stand up without the support of your hands or arms?
2. Does your lower back frequently hurt or feel stiff, particularly after exercise?
3. Do you often find yourself slouching, shoulders hunching forward, or noticing your posture is off?
4. Can you close your eyes and lift one foot off the floor without losing your balance?
5. Do you inadvertently hold your breath during exercises?
6. Does your midsection or lower back sag down while you are holding a plank position?

If you answered Yes to at least two questions, you would greatly benefit from training your core. These questions provide tell-tale signs that your core may be weak.

WHAT DOES THE QUIZ REVEAL?

1. Core strength, particularly in your abdominal area, is needed to raise yourself from a lying to a seated position as well as from a seated to a standing position. If you are relying on your hands and arms to push you up, it's because your core isn't able to do that on its own.
2. Assuming that you are not suffering from a back injury, arthritis, or recovering from surgery, pain, and stiffness in your lower back may be a lack of core strength and from weak muscles around your spine.
3. Poor posture is often an indicator of insufficient core stability.
4. Balance issues can be due to a number of factors, but many times it is from a lack of core stability. Your core muscles are the ones that stabilize you as you walk, turn, and twist.
5. Holding your breath while you exercise is an indicator that your core muscles are not as strong as they could be. Your core strength is what helps you to breathe as your body works out or engages in physical activity. The inability to both breathe and move through a core exercise at the same time signals core weakness.
6. Whether it is a straight arm or modified plank, your core is what keeps your back straight during the exercise. Any sagging in your lower body is a sign that your core isn't doing its job.

Now that we know more about the core muscles, the benefits of strengthening them, and the general state of our own cores, in the next chapter, we will look at what we can do to develop a strong core.

Key Takeaways from Chapter 1:

- ○ We can prevent the loss of muscle mass and strength that naturally occurs with aging by making a few lifestyle changes.

- ○ The core muscles in the front, sides and back of our torso support our body and our ability to do everyday activities.

- ○ A strong core gives us better balance and helps reduce pain.

Developing a Strong Core

We can't avoid age. However, we can avoid some aging. Continue to do things. Be active. Life is fantastic in the way it adjusts to demands; if you use your muscles and mind, they stay there much longer. —Charles H. Townes

Remaining strong and stable is an important part of aging well. To live an active, interesting, and fulfilling life as you enter your sixties, seventies, eighties, and beyond, you must retain the ability to perform everyday tasks. Staying physically active and maintaining core strength is important if you want to continue to do the things you enjoy.

In this chapter, we will look at the fundamentals of developing a strong core. In particular, we will learn when and where to exercise plus discover what common mistakes to avoid.

HOW TO EXERCISE YOUR CORE

Training and strengthening your core is not just performing abdominal exercises. Because your core muscles run along your entire torso from under your rib cage to your pelvis, from side to side, and along your back down to your buttocks, they take up a lot of real estate on your torso. Around thirty-five muscles, both large and small, make up your core. These muscles can be worked every day, as long as you aren't working the same ones all the time. By training a variety of these muscles, you will build a solid foundation that serves as a link between the upper and lower halves of your body. This sturdy connection allows your arms and legs to do their jobs to their fullest capacity. Let's take a look at some best practices to work on your core.

HOW TO EXERCISE YOUR CORE

Training and strengthening your core is not just performing abdominal exercises. Because your core muscles run along your entire torso from under your rib cage to your pelvis, from side to side, and along your back down to your buttocks, they take up a lot of real estate on your torso. Around thirty-five muscles, both large and small, make up your core. These muscles can be worked every day, as long as you aren't working the same ones all the time. By training a variety of these muscles, you will build a solid foundation that serves as a link between the upper and lower halves of your body. This sturdy connection allows your arms and legs to do their jobs to their fullest capacity. Let's take a look at some best practices to work on your core.

HOW TO EXERCISE YOUR CORE

Training and strengthening your core is not just performing abdominal exercises. Because your core muscles run along your entire torso from under your rib cage to your pelvis, from side to side, and along your back down to your buttocks, they take up a lot of real estate on your torso. Around thirty-five muscles, both large and small, make up your core.

These muscles can be worked every day, as long as you aren't working the same ones all the time. By training a variety of these muscles, you will build a solid foundation that serves as a link between the upper and lower halves of your body. This sturdy connection allows your arms and legs to do their jobs to their fullest capacity. Let's take a look at some best practices to work on your core.

WHEN TO EXERCISE

Some trainers recommend a morning routine, and others swear by exercising in the afternoon. What's the difference? Let's take a look.

Advantages of a morning exercise routine:

○ Consistent habit. Getting up and lacing up your sneakers each morning builds a routine that stays consistent.

○ Better sleep. Working out early helps you fall asleep and stay asleep at night.

○ Lessens hunger. You may find you are less hungry during the day if you work out in the morning.

Advantages of an afternoon exercise routine:

○ Already warmed up. Unlike exercising in the morning when your body is still waking up, and muscles are stiff, an afternoon workout happens when you are fully awake and moving about.

○ Hormone balance. Cortisol, the stress hormone, peaks in the morning but decreases as the day goes on. On the other hand, testosterone, a muscle growth hormone, is produced at higher levels in the afternoon.

Most trainers agree that exercising at night isn't the best because it can disrupt your body's circadian rhythm or internal clock. In addition, because exercise stimulates your nervous system, you may find that working out late at night may prevent you from falling or staying asleep.

Regardless of when you choose to work out, the important thing is to try to exercise consistently at the same time every day. By making regular appointments with yourself to train and strengthen your body, you will build a habit that reaps lifetime benefits.

WHERE TO EXERCISE

There are many options to choose from when deciding where to exercise. Depending on your preference, financial situation, or comfort level, you may choose to exercise in private or public. Some options of where to perform exercises include:

○ Your home. You may have a spare bedroom, space in your garage, or a spot in your backyard where you can comfortably exercise. The advantage of working out at home is the privacy and convenience of not having to go elsewhere. Plus, it's free.

You can also work out at any time of day and aren't dependent on someone else's open hours.

- ○ Gym. Whether it is a small privately-owned gym or a larger commercial gym franchise, gyms can be good places to exercise. They do have monthly fees but offer several types of cardio equipment, weight machines, free weights, and exercise classes. Many also have a trainer available to guide you through exercise routines for an additional fee. Working out at a gym can be a fun social experience and a place to connect with people.

COMMON MISTAKES TO AVOID

While core exercises aren't complicated, there are some common pitfalls to avoid. These exercises differ from those done for cardiovascular benefit, resistance training with weights, and stretching. When exercising your core, paying attention to potential mistakes when exercising your core is essential to avoid injury and discouragement.

Things to avoid when exercising your core include:

1. Poor form. Having incorrect positioning of your body, arms, or legs while performing core exercises can cause pain or injury. It also won't work the right muscles or give you the desired outcome. Poor form can sometimes be caused by the body being tired, or the exercise being too difficult.

2. Exercising too fast. Rushing through core exercises to get them done quickly will not give you the results you want. Core training requires tension and time. Doing the exercises slowly and correctly is the goal.

3. Doing too much too soon. We all want results, and we want them right now. So, we jump in and do too much too soon! Start at a reasonable pace and add time and difficulty slowly. If you get too sore or injure yourself, you may become discouraged and quit altogether.

Before we get to the exciting part, please accept my heartfelt gratitude for downloading my book. Please leave a review on Amazon to let me know what you think of the book so far(You can always change this after reading the whole book). This will benefit a lot of other individuals who are looking for a book like mine. To me, that would be really valuable.

Scan The QR Code to Leave a Review:

I sincerely hope that this book proves to be an invaluable asset for you as you navigate the challenges of restoring and preserving stability, with the ultimate goal of preventing falls and enhancing your overall health.

We will learn the best mat, seated, and standing core exercises, in the following few chapters. Let's get the exercises started!

Mat Core Exercises

Don't go through life, grow through life. —*Eric Butterworth*

Mat exercises are an effective way to train and strengthen your core. Most people associate mat core exercises with old-fashioned sit-ups or crunches. While sit-ups may have some merit, they aren't the best exercise for us as we get older. Sit-ups and crunches can put unnecessary strain on our spine, backs, and necks. The mat exercises outlined in this chapter concentrate on training your core while close to the floor. As you might have guessed, there is no fear of falling or losing your balance while doing these mat exercises, so they are perfect for those who may suffer from instability issues or have trouble standing or sitting. These exercises make it convenient for you to work out your core from an all-fours or reclined position. You will need a padded mat or carpeted floor to perform these.

BIRD DOG

Time per rep: 20 seconds   **Total time: 3 minutes**

How to:

1. Place hands and knees on the floor, ensuring that your hands are directly below your shoulders and knees directly below your hips.

2. Raise your right knee off the floor and extend your right foot back and up off the floor until it is parallel to the floor, if possible.

3. Now, raise your left hand off the floor and extend it out in front of you. Protect your neck by continuing to look at the floor. Take a deep breath in and slowly exhale.

4. Slowly bring your knee and hand back to starting position. Repeat two more times.

5. Do the opposite side by raising your left knee and right hand off the floor. Repeat twice.

Level Up:

You can make this exercise more challenging. When your knee and opposite hand are extended out, slowly bring that knee and opposite elbow together below you, exhaling as you do so. Do the same with the other side.

Take Note:

If this exercise causes you to lose your balance, keep both hands on the floor as you raise your leg. Alternatively, you can keep both knees on the floor as you raise your hand. Your core will strengthen over time.

BRIDGE

Time per rep: 15 seconds   **Total time: 2 minutes**

How to:

1. Lie on your back on the mat. Bend your knees so that your feet are flat on the floor and knees are pointed towards the ceiling.

2. Place your feet about hip-width apart. Tighten your buttocks and abdominals as you slowly raise your hips straight up and off the floor. Your knees, hips, and shoulders should form a diagonal line.

3. Hold the raised position for two breaths in and out, then gently lower your hips back down to the floor.

4. Repeat three more times.

Level Up:

To make this exercise more challenging, hold the raised bridge position for 30 seconds.

Take Note:

If you have any neck or spinal pain, check with your doctor and be extra cautious doing this exercise.

DEAD BUG

Time per rep: 20 seconds   **Total time: 3 minutes**

How to:

1. Lie down with your back on the floor. Bend your knees and lift your feet off the floor so that your knees are directly over your hips.

2. Raise your feet so that your shins are parallel to the floor. Press the small of your back into the floor as you tighten your abdominals.

3. Lift both arms towards the ceiling with palms facing each other.

4. Keeping your knees bent, inhale and slowly lower your right foot until your toes touch the floor. Exhale and bring your foot back up to starting position.

5. Alternate doing the left foot and right foot, five times each.

Level Up:

Once you are comfortable with this exercise, you can make it more challenging by adding the arms. As you lower one foot, also lower the opposite arm by reaching with your hand back above your head. Exhale as you return the foot and hand to the starting position. Alternate by doing the other hand and foot.

Take Note:

Don't arch your back while doing this exercise. Instead, keep your tummy firm and the small of your back pressed into the floor.

MODIFIED CURL UP

Time per rep: 20 seconds   **Total time: 3 minutes**

How to:

1. Lie down with your back on the mat. Bend both knees so that they are pointing to the ceiling and feet are flat on the floor.

2. Place your hands, palms down, between the floor and the small of your back. This will help protect your back.

3. Slowly straighten your right leg and extend your foot until the heel touches the floor. Keep your other leg bent.

4. Tighten your abdominals as you raise your head and shoulders slightly off the floor. Only raise them by one or two inches, this is not a large lift. Hold for five seconds and slowly lower back down.

5. Repeat the move three more times.

6. Switch legs. Straighten your left leg and extend your foot while keeping your other leg bent. Tighten your core as you raise your head and shoulders off the mat. Lower back down and repeat three more times.

Level Up:

To make this more difficult, hold the lift for 10 seconds.

Take Note:

Be aware of your neck position while lifting your head and shoulders. Do not bend your neck forward to lift higher. Instead, keep your shoulders, neck, and head in a straight line.

MOUNTAIN CLIMBER

Time per rep: 15 seconds   **Total time: 2 minutes**

How to:

1. Start from a kneeling position with your hands and knees on the mat.

2. Lift your knees from the mat and extend your legs straight behind you. Your hands should be directly under your shoulders and feet about hip-width apart with toes touching the mat.

3. From this plank position, tighten your abdominals and exhale as you bend your right knee and bring it up towards the middle of your chest. Inhale as you return your leg to the starting position.

4. Switch legs and exhale as you bend your left knee, bringing it towards the middle of your chest. Return your leg to the starting position.

5. Continue to do the mountain climbers, switching legs each time, for three more times on each leg.

Level Up:

Add more repetitions as your core becomes stronger, working your way up to 10 or 12 times on each side.

Take Note:

Keep your eyes on the floor and don't let your head drop. Keep your neck long and in a straight line with your head and shoulders.

PLANK

Time per rep: 20 seconds   **Total time: 2 minutes**

How to:

1. Start from a kneeling position with your hands and knees on the mat.

2. Lift your knees from the mat and extend your legs out straight behind you. Your hands should be directly under your shoulders and feet about hip-width apart, with toes touching the mat.

3. Hold this plank position for 10 seconds. Lower knees to the floor and rest a few seconds. Repeat the plank three or four more times.

4. If this is too hard, try a modified plank. Instead of lifting both knees off the floor, only do one knee at a time.

Level Up:

As you get stronger, hold the plank position for longer periods. Work up to 30 seconds, then one minute.

Take Note:

Pay attention to your lower back. Don't let it arch, but rather keep it in a straight line with your shoulders and hips.

SEGMENTAL ROTATION

Time per rep: 20 seconds   **Total time: 2 minutes**

How to:

1. Lie down with your back on the floor.

2. Bend both knees so they are pointing to the ceiling, and both feet are on the floor. Extend both arms out from your sides, palms facing the floor.

3. Slowly lower both bent knees to the right side. Your upper body should face the ceiling, and only your lower body moves. You may be able to have your right knee lower all the way to the floor, but if you can't, that is okay. Only lower as far as you feel comfortable. It should not be painful.

4. Inhale, tighten your abdominals, and exhale as you raise both knees back to the starting position.

5. Doing the other side, lower both bent knees to the left as far as is comfortable. Bring both knees back to starting position.

6. Repeat the exercise on both sides three more times.

Level Up:

As a variation, you can move your head and look in the opposite direction of your knees. If your knees are lowered to the right, rotate your head and look to the left. You will feel a gentle stretch on the right side of your neck. When your knees are lowered to the left, look right.

Take Note:

Keep your eyes on the floor and don't let your head drop. Keep your neck long and in a straight line with your head and shoulders.

SIDE PLANK

Time per rep: 20 seconds   **Total time: 2 minutes**

How to:

1. Lie on the floor on your right side. Extend your legs, so they are straight, with hips stacked one on top of the other.
2. Bring your right arm under you. Prop up your upper body by placing your right forearm on the floor directly under your right shoulder. Be sure your right forearm and hand are placed on the floor for support.
3. Tighten your core and raise your hips up and off the floor. Your feet, knees, hips, and shoulders should form a straight diagonal line. Breathing normally, hold for five seconds.
4. Slowly lower hip back down to the floor. Rest a few seconds, then repeat the side plank three more times.
5. Switch to your left side. Doing the same thing on this side, extend your legs and bring your left arm under you. Raise your hips off the floor to form a diagonal line and hold for five seconds. Lower and repeat three more times.
6. If this exercise is too hard, try doing it with your bottom leg bent and resting on the floor instead.

Level Up:

Once five seconds is easy for you, increase your time to 10 or 20 seconds on each side. To make this exercise even more challenging, you can do it with your bottom hand on the floor and your arm fully extended. You will be supporting yourself with your hand rather than your forearm.

Take Note:

Don't let your hips droop down. Keep the diagonal line from your feet, knees, hips, and shoulders.

SIDE PLANK WITH ROTATION

Time per rep: 20 seconds   **Total time: 2 minutes**

How to:

1. Get into a side plank position, lying on your right side with legs extended, hips stacked, and right forearm on the floor supporting you.

2. Tighten your core muscles as you lift your hips off the floor.

3. Extend your left arm up towards the ceiling and inhale.

4. Exhale and bring your left arm down and under your right ribs.

5. Return your left arm up and extend it towards the ceiling.

6. Slowly lower your hips to the floor. Repeat the sequence three more times.

7. Switch sides by lying on your left side. Lift your hips off the floor and now extend your right arm to the ceiling, bring it down under your left ribs, and extend up again. Lower your hips and repeat three more times.

Level Up:

You can change the intensity of this exercise. To make it easier, keep your bottom leg bent and resting on the floor. To make it more challenging, support yourself with your hand and a straight arm instead of your forearm.

Take Note:

Keep your gaze straight ahead in front of you. If your balance is good, your eyes and head can follow your moving arm as it goes underneath you.

SINGLE-LEG ABDOMINAL PRESS

Time per rep: 20 seconds   **Total time: 2 minutes**

How to:

1. Lie on the mat on your back. Bend both knees so that they are pointing towards the ceiling, and your feet are flat on the floor.

2. Raise your right leg and foot so that your shin is parallel to the floor. Your knee should be at a 90-degree angle.

3. Tighten your abdominals as you place your right hand on your right knee and try to press it away from you. At the same time, have your right knee resist against your hand. Hold for five seconds, then lower your leg to the starting position. Repeat on this side three more times.

4. Switch legs. Raise your left leg and foot, forming a 90-degree angle. With your left hand, press your left knee away from you while trying to resist with your knee. Repeat on this side three more times.

Level Up:

To make this more challenging, raise both knees simultaneously. Press both hands against both knees as they resist.

Take Note:

Keep your back in a neutral position. Neither arch your lower back nor press it into the floor.

SUPERMAN

Time per rep: 20 seconds   **Total time: 2 minutes**

How to:

1. Lie on the floor, face down, with arms overhead and legs extended out straight.

2. Inhale, tighten your core muscles, and while exhaling, simultaneously raise your chest, arms, and legs off the floor a few inches. Hold the position for five seconds, then slowly lower back down to the floor. Repeat six times.

3. To make this exercise easier, you can choose to raise only your chest and arms off the floor. Or raise only your legs off the floor.

Level Up:

Make this exercise more challenging by making small flutter or paddling motions while your arms and legs are lifted.

Take Note:

If your hips need extra support, place a folded towel under them. You can also place one under your forehead.

SUPINE TOE TAPS

Time per rep: 15 seconds   **Total time: 2 minutes**

How to:

1. Lie down with your back on a mat. Bend your knees so they face the ceiling and feet are flat on the mat. Rest arms at your side with palms facing down.

2. Slowly raise both feet up off the mat so that your shins are now parallel to the floor and knees are at a 90-degree angle.

3. Keeping your right knee bent, lower your right foot to the floor until your toes touch. Bring the foot back up.

4. Now do the same with your left foot, tapping the floor with your left toes and bringing it back up.

5. Alternate feet, doing a total of four toe taps per foot.

Level Up:

Increase the number of toe taps as your core gets stronger. To make this harder, do both feet at the same time.

Take Note:

Don't arch your back while performing this exercise. If your lower back needs extra support, place your hands or a small, folded towel under the small of your back.

Seated Core
Exercises

Life isn't about finding yourself. Life is about creating yourself. —*George Bernard Shaw*

You may be surprised to learn that seated exercises are an effective way to strengthen your core. Seated exercising is a low-impact and safe way to work your core and get in some cardio movement and strength training. If you have suffered from a stroke, fall, or another challenge that has weakened your core, seated exercises are a smart way to regain your strength and balance. It also lessens the likelihood of falling. Seated exercises are perfect for those who find it challenging to get down and up from the floor, those who are disabled and require a wheelchair, or those who have balance and stability issues. These seated exercises can help you regain and maintain a strong core and will help build your confidence and abilities to perform daily tasks.

In this chapter, we will look at twelve of the best seated exercises for your core. For these seated exercises, it is recommended to sit in a sturdy, straight-backed chair with no arms. If you need extra stability, place the chair near a table or low counter that you can place your hand upon if required.

BAND EXTENSION

Time per rep: 15 seconds   **Total time: 2 minutes**

How to:

1. Loop a resistance band around the back of a sturdy chair.

2. Sit down in the chair. Place your hands in the handles and loop the band around your hands until the band is taut when your hands are resting in your lap.

3. Sit up tall with your feet flat on the floor. With arms bent, lift both hands to the same height as your belly button.

4. Tighten your core muscles. Push your hands out straight in front of you until your arms are fully extended. You should feel resistance from the band. Hold for five seconds, then bend arms and return your hands to your lap.

5. Repeat seven more times.

Level Up:

If you don't have a resistance band, you can use three-pound weights in each hand instead. There won't be resistance, but your core muscles will still be exercised.

Take Note:

Don't slouch or hunch up while doing this exercise. Sit up tall and keep your shoulders relaxed and down.

HALF ROLLBACKS

Time per rep: 15 seconds   **Total time: 2 minutes**

How to:

1. Sit erect in a chair with your feet flat on the floor and knees bent.

2. Lift both arms out in front of you with your elbows bent, fingertips touching, and palms facing towards you.

3. Slowly round your shoulders and upper back as you contract your abdominals and look down at your thighs. Hold for five seconds, then slowly roll back up. Once returned to the starting position, reset your shoulders by shrugging them up, back, and down.

4. Repeat the exercise seven more times.

Level Up:

You can make this slightly more difficult. Instead of having your feet flat on the floor while seated, raise your heels so that only your toes are touching the floor.

Take Note:

It's natural to hold your breath while performing this exercise. Remember to breathe normally.

LEG TAPS

Time per rep: 15 seconds   **Total time: 2 minutes**

How to:

1. Sit upright in a chair or on a bench with your knees bent. Sit closer towards the edge but with your buttocks still on the seat.

2. With feet flat on the floor, place your hands on the seat of the chair for support.

3. Extend both legs out straight in front of you with feet still touching the floor. Tighten up your abdominals as you lift both feet off the floor a few inches. Hold for five seconds and slowly lower back down to the floor.

4. Repeat three more times.

Level Up:

To increase the difficulty, you can hold your feet off the floor for 10 seconds, then 20 seconds.

Take Note:

Be sure not to hunch up your shoulders or lean too far back when you raise your legs up. Try to maintain an upright position.

RESISTED KNEE LIFT

Time per rep: 15 seconds   **Total time: 1 minutes**

How to:

1. Sit upright in a chair or on a bench with your knees bent. Sit closer towards the edge but with your buttocks still on the seat.

2. With feet flat on the floor, place your hands on the seat of the chair for support.

3. Extend both legs out straight in front of you with feet still touching the floor. Tighten up your abdominals as you lift both feet off the floor a few inches. Hold for five seconds and slowly lower back down to the floor.

4. Repeat three more times.

Level Up:

You can make this harder by lifting both legs at the same time while pressing down on them with both hands.

Take Note:

Maintain good posture while doing this move.

SEATED DEAD BUG

Time per rep: 10 seconds　　　　　　　　　**Total time: 1 minutes**

How to:

1. Sit erect in a chair. Your knees should be bent and your feet flat on the floor.

2. Raise both arms straight out in front of you.

3. Inhale. As you exhale, tighten your tummy and lift your right arm up above your head. Bring your arm back down so it is straight out in front of you.

4. Switch arms. This time lift your left arm above your head while tightening your abs. Return the arm to the starting position.

5. Repeat on both arms five more times.

Level Up:

To increase the difficulty, raise the opposite foot off the floor as you bring your arm up above your head.

Take Note:

It's tempting to do this exercise quickly and wind up pumping your arms up and down. Remember to move through the exercise slowly and deliberately while keeping your tummy tightened.

SEATED FORWARD ROLL-UP

Time per rep: 15 seconds   **Total time: 2 minutes**

How to:

1. Sit up tall in a chair. Extend both legs out in front of you with your heels on the floor and toes pointed to the ceiling.

2. Raise your arms straight out in front of you.

3. Tuck your chin in towards your chest as you roll forward with your arms extended. Your hands should be reaching towards your toes.

4. Tighten your abs and slowly roll back up to the starting position.

5. Repeat the exercise seven more times.

Level Up:

Once you are comfortable with this exercise, you can increase the difficulty. Take twice as long to roll back up as you did to roll down.

Take Note:

Be sure to do these moves slowly, so you don't use any momentum as you roll down or up.

SEATED JUMPING JACKS

Time per rep: 10 seconds   **Total time: 2 minutes**

How to:

1. Sit erect in a chair with your knees bent. Have your feet on the floor but with your heels slightly lifted. Hands are down on either side of you.

2. Tighten your abs as you raise both hands up above your head. Simultaneously lift both feet off the floor and out to the sides like you would for a standing jumping jack. Bring hands and feet back to starting position.

3. Repeat the exercise five more times.

4. If you find this to be too hard, do the seated jumping jacks one side at a time. Instead of lifting both arms and both legs, just do the left arm and left leg. Switch to the other leg and repeat.

Level Up:

This exercise can also count as cardio when 30 or more jumping jacks are done. For those who have knee or hip pain, this is a low-impact way to do jumping jacks.

Take Note:

Don't allow your neck to crane forward or your upper back to hunch while completing these moves. Keep your neck and upper back neutral and relaxed.

SEATED LEG LIFT

Time per rep: 15 seconds   **Total time: 2 minutes**

How to:

1. With both feet flat on the floor, sit in a chair with your knees bent. Place your hands on either side of the chair seat for support.

2. Straighten your right leg while keeping your foot on the floor. Tighten your tummy as you raise your right foot off the floor until it is parallel to the floor, if possible. Hold the position for five seconds, then slowly lower your foot back to the floor.

3. Reset by sitting with both knees bent. Switch to the other side by straightening your left leg. Raise your left foot and hold for five seconds before lowering back down.

4. Repeat each leg three more times.

Level Up:

As a variation, you can concentrate on one leg at a time. Do all six reps with one leg before switching to the other instead of alternating legs.

Take Note:

Be sure not to slouch or round your back as you lift your leg.

SEATED RUSSIAN TWIST

Time per rep: 10 seconds   **Total time: 1 minutes**

How to:

1. Sit erect in a chair with your knees bent. Have your feet on the floor but with your heels slightly lifted. Hands are down on either side of you.

2. Tighten your abs as you raise both hands up above your head. Simultaneously lift both feet off the floor and out to the sides like you would for a standing jumping jack. Bring hands and feet back to starting position.

3. Repeat the exercise five more times.

4. If you find this to be too hard, do the seated jumping jacks one side at a time. Instead of lifting both arms and both legs, just do the left arm and left leg. Switch to the other leg and repeat.

Level Up:

This exercise can also count as cardio when 30 or more jumping jacks are done. For those who have knee or hip pain, this is a low-impact way to do jumping jacks.

Take Note:

Don't allow your neck to crane forward or your upper back to hunch while completing these moves. Keep your neck and upper back neutral and relaxed.

SEATED LEG LIFT

Time per rep: 15 seconds   **Total time: 2 minutes**

How to:

1. With both feet flat on the floor, sit in a chair with your knees bent. Place your hands on either side of the chair seat for support.

2. Straighten your right leg while keeping your foot on the floor. Tighten your tummy as you raise your right foot off the floor until it is parallel to the floor, if possible. Hold the position for five seconds, then slowly lower your foot back to the floor.

3. Reset by sitting with both knees bent. Switch to the other side by straightening your left leg. Raise your left foot and hold for five seconds before lowering back down.

4. Repeat each leg three more times.

Level Up:

As a variation, you can concentrate on one leg at a time. Do all six reps with one leg before switching to the other instead of alternating legs.

Take Note:

Be sure not to slouch or round your back as you lift your leg.

SEATED RUSSIAN TWIST

Time per rep: 10 seconds   **Total time: 1 minutes**

How to:

1. Sit up tall in a chair. Your knees should be bent and your feet on the floor with your heels slightly lifted.

2. Bend your elbows at a 90-degree angle with your hands in front of you. Clasp your hands together, interlocking your fingers.

3. Tighten your abs as you move your clasped hands to the outside of your right leg, then slowly move your hands to the outside of your left leg. Allow your eyes, head, and shoulders to follow the movement of your hands. Breathe normally throughout.

4. Repeat the exercise seven more times.

Level Up:

Increase the difficulty by lifting your feet completely off the floor as you twist from side to side.

Take Note:

This should be a slow, continuous movement as you move your hands from side to side. Take care not to jerk your hands over as you change sides.

SEATED TWIST

Time per rep: 20 seconds   **Total time: 2 minutes**

How to:

1. Sit in a chair with your feet flat on the floor.

2. Raise your arms and hands straight out in front of you so that your hands are at eye level.

3. Tighten your core as you move your hands and arms to the right while gently twisting your torso. Hands should still be at eye level. Hold the twist for five seconds. The rotation should stem from your midsection, not just your shoulders. Slowly return to starting position with arms straight ahead.

4. Now twist to the other side by bringing your arms to the left while twisting your midsection. Hold for five seconds before returning to the starting position.

5. Repeat the exercise five more times.

Level Up:

To make this exercise more challenging, hold a three to five-pound weight while doing the twists.

Take Note:

Check with your doctor before doing this or any twisting exercise if you have osteoporosis or have recently had back surgery.

SIDE BENDS

Time per rep: 15 seconds   **Total time: 1 minutes**

How to:

1. Sit in a chair and maintain good posture. Knees should be bent, and feet flat on the floor. Let your arms hang down on either side of your body.

2. Take a breath in and as you exhale, lower your right arm towards the floor as you bend sideways at the waist. Using your core muscles, slowly come back up to the starting position.

3. Switch to the other side by lowering your left arm to the floor as you exhale and bend sideways to the left. Slowly return to the starting position.

4. Repeat exercise five more times.

Level Up:

Add some resistance by holding three-pound weights in each hand as you do the side bends.

Take Note:

Take care that your chest is facing forward as you bend at the waist. Don't allow your chest to twist and face the floor.

SINGLE KNEE TUCK

Time per rep: 20 seconds   **Total time: 2 minutes**

How to:

1. Sit up tall. Come closer to the edge of the chair but still have both buttocks fully on the seat. Be sure your knees are bent, and feet are flat on the floor.

2. Grip the sides of the seat with both hands for support.

3. Keeping your knee bent, raise your right knee until it is higher than your hip, if possible. Hold it up for five seconds as you keep your abs tight. Lower your leg back down to the starting position.

4. Switch legs, this time lifting your left knee and holding for five seconds. Lower the leg back down.

5. Repeat five more times.

Level Up:

To make this more challenging, lift both knees at the same time.

Take Note:

Be sure not to lean back as you lift your knees. Maintain an upright posture.

Standing Core Exercises

Aging gracefully means being flexible, being open, allowing change, enjoying change and loving yourself. — Wendy Whelan

Can you exercise your core while you are standing? You can! Performing core exercises from a standing position provides a change from how core exercises are traditionally done and provides some fresh moves for core muscle training. Surprising your muscles causes them to be stimulated and grow due to the change in position and type of exercise. You can keep your muscles guessing by not doing the same old same old. Standing exercises require a little more balance and stability on your feet. Use a sturdy chair or nearby countertop for extra support.

CORE ROTATION

Time per rep: 10 seconds   **Total time: 1 minutes**

How to:

1. Stand up tall. Have your knees slightly bent and your feet hip-width distance apart and flat on the floor.

2. Bend your arms at the elbows to form a 90-degree angle with your hands out in front of you.

3. Keeping your abdominals tight, bend your torso over to the right, bend forward, then bend to the left. This should be a smooth arc going from the right side to the left side.

4. Do the same thing but going in the other direction. Bend your torso over to the left, forward, and right in a smooth movement while keeping your abs tight.

5. Repeat five more times.

Level Up:

To add difficulty to this move, hold a three or five-pound weight with both hands.

Take Note:

It's easy to hold your breath as you concentrate on your abs. Keep breathing normally throughout this exercise

FIGURE 8 ROW

Time per rep: 10 seconds   **Total time: 1 minutes**

How to:

1. Stand comfortably with feet hip-width distance apart and flat on the floor. Knees can be slightly bent.

2. Raise both arms and bend at your elbows. Place one hand under the opposite elbow and let the other hand rest on top of the other elbow. Your forearms should be resting one on top of the other at chest height.

3. Keep your posture upright as you tighten your ab muscles and move your right elbow down towards your right hip. Bring your right elbow up to shoulder height.

4. Work the other side by moving your left elbow down to your left hip, then up to shoulder height. Your elbows should be drawing a figure-eight in the air in front of you.

5. Repeat the move, alternating side, five more times.

Level Up:

If you have shoulder pain or it is difficult for you to stack one forearm on top of the other, an option is to hold your hands out in front of you with elbows at a 90-degree angle. Make a fist with both hands with palms down and knuckles up. Do the figure-eight motion now. It will mimic paddling a canoe, minus the oar.

Take Note:

Don't let your torso hunch over too far to the right or left. Maintain an upright posture and let your abs do the work.

KNEE ROTATION

Time per rep: 10 seconds   **Total time: 2 minutes**

How to:

1. Stand up tall with both feet flat on the floor and hip-width distance apart.

2. Clasp both hands together in front of you with elbows bent at a 90-degree angle.

3. Bring your hands over to the right side of your waist and let your torso twist to the right.

4. Now, bring your hands to the left side and twist your torso to the left. Simultaneously, lift your left knee and foot as your torso twists to the left.

5. Bring your left knee down as you twist back to the right side.

6. Repeat this same side five more times.

7. Switch sides by starting with your hands over on the left side of your waist and twisting your torso to the left. As you bring your hands over the right and twist to the right, raise your right knee. Repeat on this side five more times.

Level Up:

If you can't lift your entire foot off the floor without losing your balance, you can modify this move by just lifting your heel off the floor while keeping your toes connected to the floor.

Take Note:

Remember to keep your core muscles engaged throughout this exercise; otherwise, you are just twisting!

KNEE TUCK EXTENSION

Time per rep: 10 seconds   **Total time: 2 minutes**

How to:

1. Stand up tall with feet hip-width distance apart. If you need a sturdy chair or countertop to hold on to for balance, stand next to that.

2. Stretch your right arm up overhead and inhale. As you exhale, bend your arm and bring your elbow down. At the same time, raise your right knee and try to have your elbow and knee touch. Your left hand can rest on your waist or on a chair.

3. Repeat five more times.

4. Switch sides. Now stretch your left arm overhead and bring your left elbow down as you bring your left knee up to meet it. Repeat five more times on this side.

Level Up:

To increase the difficulty, bend both arms and place your hands behind your head. Facing straight ahead, bend your torso to the right as you bring your right elbow and knee towards each other. Do the same thing on the left.

Take Note:

You are bringing your elbow and knee towards each other. It's okay if they don't touch.

SIDE BENDS

Time per rep: 10 seconds   **Total time: 2 minutes**

How to:

1. Stand erect with your feet at hip-width distance apart and feet flat on the floor.

2. Bend your left arm at the elbow with your left hand out in front of you so that your left elbow forms a 90-degree angle. Let your right arm hang straight down at your right side.

3. Keeping your chest and head looking straight ahead, tighten your abs as you bend your torso to the right so that your right hand slides down your right side towards your right knee. Return to the starting position. Repeat five more times.

4. Switch sides by bending your right elbow and having your left arm down by your side. Bend your torso to the left and allow your left hand to slide down your left side. Return to the starting position, then repeat five more times.

Level Up:

Adding two or three-pound hand weights will make this exercise more challenging. Take care not to add too heavy of a weight.

Take Note:

Don't let your chest collapse as you bend to the side. Keep your chest out and facing straight ahead.

SQUAT

Time per rep: 10 seconds   **Total time: 1 minutes**

How to:

1. Stand with your feet hip-width distance apart.
2. Raise both arms straight out in front of you as you bend your knees.
3. Squat as low as is comfortable and hold for five seconds. Return to standing.
4. Repeat the exercise five more times.

Level Up:

You can make this more challenging by doing more squats. Try to do 10 in a row, then 20, and increase from there.

Take Note:

Squats work on your core muscles in your lower back, pelvis, and glutes. If you have balancing issues, be sure to hold on to a sturdy chair or countertop.

STANDING BICYCLE CRUNCH

Time per rep: 10 seconds   **Total time: 2 minutes**

How to:

1. Stand up tall with feet hip-width distance apart and knees slightly bent.

2. Have a sturdy chair or countertop next to you for balance. Bend your right arm and place your right hand behind your head.

3. Bend your left knee and lift your left foot off the floor. Twist your torso to bring your right elbow towards your raised left knee. Return to the starting position.

4. Repeat the exercise on this side five more times.

5. Switch sides. Place your left hand behind your head and lift your right foot off the floor. Twist to the right as you bring your left elbow to your right knee. Repeat five times.

Level Up:

If you don't have stability challenges, try doing this without holding on to anything. Place both hands behind your head as you do the standing crunches, alternating from one knee to the other.

Take Note:

Be sure you are not pulling on your neck or bending it too far forward as you move through your crunches.

STANDING BIRD DOG

Time per rep: 10 seconds   **Total time: 2 minutes**

How to:

1. Stand up tall with your feet hip-width distance apart, and arms by your sides.

2. Stand next to a sturdy chair or countertop to hold on to for balance. Raise your right hand straight above your head while at the same time raising your left knee and left foot off the floor. Hold this pose for five seconds, then return to the starting position.

3. Repeat this side five more times.

4. Switch sides by raising your left hand above your head while raising the opposite knee. Repeat five more times.

Level Up:

Add a balance challenge to this exercise by not holding on to anything.

Take Note:

Moving slowly through this exercise and contracting your core muscles will ensure that you are working them.

STANDING CRUNCH

Time per rep: 10 seconds   **Total time: 1 minutes**

How to:

1. Stand with feet about hip-width distance apart and knees slightly bent.

2. Bend your elbows so that your hands are out in front of you and elbows are at a 90-degree angle.

3. Inhale. As you exhale, tighten your core, and slowly bend forward at the waist. Bend forward as far as you can comfortably, but don't go lower than your belly button. Slowly return to a standing position.

4. Repeat five more times.

Level Up:

As a variation, you can raise your hands and place them behind your head as you would for regular sit-ups. Be sure not to pull on your neck.

Take Note:

Keep your shoulders relaxed as you move through this exercise. Don't allow them to hunch up.

TWIST

Time per rep: 10 seconds   **Total time: 1 minutes**

How to:

1. With feet about hip-width distance apart and feet flat on the floor, stand up tall.
2. Bend your arms at the elbow with your hands in front of you so that elbows form a 90-degree angle.
3. Keeping your hips straight ahead, tighten your abs and twist your torso and arms turning to the right.
4. Come back to the starting point and twist your torso and arms turning to the left.
5. Repeat the moves five more times.

Level Up:

To increase the difficulty, hold a two or three-pound weight in each hand.

Take Note:

Don't swing from side to side using momentum. This should be a slow, deliberate twist from the waist up. Keep your feet stationary.

WIDE SIDE CRUNCH

Time per rep: 10 seconds   **Total time: 2 minutes**

How to:

1. Stand with your feet wide apart, and toes slightly pointed out. Bend your knees as far as is comfortable or until thighs are almost parallel with the floor.

2. Bend both arms and place your hands behind your head.

3. Keep your chest facing straight ahead, bend your torso and upper body over to the right. Your right elbow should be reaching down towards your right thigh. Return to center. Repeat five more times.

4. Now bend your torso and upper body over to the left with your left elbow pointing down towards your left thigh. Return to center and repeat five more times.

Level Up:

Instead of doing one side at a time, alternate bending to the right and then to the left.

Take Note:

Don't pull on your neck or hunch forward as you do this exercise.

WOOD CHOPS

Time per rep: 10 seconds   **Total time: 1 minutes**

How to:

1. Standing upright with your feet flat on the floor, have a slight bend in your knees.

2. Interlock your fingers as you clasp your hands together. Bring your hands up to, or slightly above, your right shoulder.

3. In one motion, bring your clasped hands down from your right shoulder to the opposite hip. Keep your core tight and engaged as you do this. Repeat five more times.

4. Switch sides by bringing your clasped hands up towards your left shoulder. Move your hands from your left shoulder down to the opposite hip in a single motion. Repeat five more times.

Level Up:

If you have had a shoulder injury or surgery, it may be uncomfortable to have both hands clasped together in this exercise. A variation is to only use one hand. Bring your right hand from your right shoulder down to your opposite hip and vice versa.

Take Note:

Don't allow your hips to move from side to side. Keep them as stationary as possible.

Core Exercises with a Partner

I get by with a little help from my friends. —*The Beatles*

Working out with a spouse, partner, helper, or workout buddy is fun and encouraging. It makes the time go quicker and gives us an extra incentive to complete our exercises together. Pick a workout partner that is encouraging, motivated, and consistent. Some of the partner exercises require a bit more strength, but with time and practice, you will be able to do these easily.

HAND SHADOWING

Time per rep: Varies   **Total time: 2 minutes**

How to:

1. Stand face-to-face with your partner. Your feet should be hip-width apart, and knees slightly bent.

2. You and your partner will bend your right arms with elbows at a 90-degree angle. Allow the backs of your hands to touch and firmly press them together.

3. Keeping the backs of you and your partner's hands pressed together in line with the center of your bodies, try to press your partner's hand away as they resist. Move your hand up and down, still trying to press their hand away. Continue for one minute.

Level Up:

As a variation, you can press your palms together instead of the backs of your hands.

Take Note:

Tighten your abs each time you move or press your partner's hand.

LEG RAISE PUSH DOWN

Time per rep: 10 seconds   **Total time: 1 minutes**

How to:

1. You will lie down on your back on a mat that is on the floor. Your partner will stand with their feet just above your head and facing towards your legs.

2. Raise your arms above your head and, with both hands, grab the outside of their ankles for support.

3. Lift both of your feet off the floor. Bring them up so that they are straight up above your hips. Keep your legs straight or with a slight bend.

4. With their hands, your partner will push both of your feet away. As your feet fall towards the floor, tighten your abdominal muscles to prevent them from reaching the floor and bring them back up above your hips.

5. Your partner will push your feet down again, and you will bring them back up again five more times.

Level Up:

If this is too difficult, start off doing one leg at a time. As you get stronger, you can work your way up to doing both legs together.

Take Note:

Don't let your lower back arch too much. Try to keep it relaxed but taut.

PARTNER GET UP

Time per rep: 15 seconds   **Total time: 1 minutes**

How to:

1. Lie down on a mat with your knees bent and pointing towards the ceiling. Your partner stands at your feet, facing you.

2. Raise both arms as your partner grabs both of your hands.

3. Using your ab muscles, sit up. Still holding on to your partner's hands, raise yourself up from sitting to standing.

4. Repeat three more times.

Level Up:

To make this more difficult, use only one hand. With your right hand, grab your partner's left hand as you sit up and stand up.

Take Note:

If you are using only one hand, be sure to do an equal number of moves with the other hand, too.

PARTNER HEEL TAP

Time per rep: 10 seconds   **Total time: 1 minutes**

How to:

1. Lie down on your back on a mat. Your partner will stand with their feet at your head, facing your legs and feet.

2. Loop a resistance band under your feet and bend your knees, so they are pointing towards the ceiling. Your partner will grab the handles of the resistance band.

3. As your partner holds the handles of the band, keep your knees bent and lower your heels to the floor. You will feel your abdominals contract. Once you tap your heels, return your legs to the starting position.

4. Repeat five more times

Level Up:

As a variation, you can do one leg at a time. Loop the band under one foot as you lower that one to the floor.

Take Note:

Take care that the band is looped under the middle of your foot (not just looped at the ball of your feet) so that it doesn't slip off and snap towards you or your partner.

PARTNER PUSH

Time per rep: Varies   **Total time: 1 minutes**

How to:

1. Stand tall, facing your partner. Both of you bend your right arms so that your elbows are at a 90-degree angle. With fingers facing up towards the ceiling, press your right palms together.

2. Both of you take a slight step back with your right foot so that your left foot is in front.

3. With right palms pressing towards each other, slowly push your partner's hand back as they gently resist until their hand is almost in line with their chest.

4. Now your partner will slowly push your hand back towards your chest as you resist. Keep going back and forth on this hand for one minute.

5. Switch sides. Do the same exercise with the palms of your left hands pressing against each other. Repeat going back and forth for one minute.

Level Up:

As you get stronger, your partner can resist more strongly against your push.

Take Note:

Remember to tighten your tummy as you push against each other's palms.

PARTNER SQUAT USING BOTH HANDS

Time per rep: 10 seconds　　　　　　　　**Total time: 1 minutes**

How to:

1. Stand upright facing your partner, a few feet apart, with your feet hip-width apart.

2. Grab both hands with your partner. At the same time, both of you lower into a squat. Go as low as is comfortable, then return to standing.

3. Repeat five more times.

Level Up:

To make this harder, only hang on with one hand. Both of you grab each other's right hands and lower into a squat. Be sure to switch sides and do the exercise with your left hands.

Take Note:

You may find that you can squat a little lower with a partner because of the counterweight balance they provide.

REACH AND TOUCH PLANK

Time per rep: 10 seconds   **Total time: 1 minutes**

How to:

1. Both you and your partner get into a plank position on the mat, facing each other. Your heads should be close and your feet away from each other.

2. You and your partner lift your right hands and touch each other's left shoulder. Alternatively, you can touch each other's right hand. Return to the starting position.

3. Switch sides and lift your left hands and touch each other.

4. Keep switching back and forth until one minute is up.

Level Up:

Depending on your strength, you can do this plank on your knees (a modified plank) or on your toes (regular plank).

Take Note:

To keep your balance, place your feet slightly wider than normal for extra stability.

Warm-Up and Cool Down

I love laugh lines. It means you've had a good life. —Aerin Lauder

People often forget to warm-up their bodies before doing any exercise. Taking five minutes to get your blood moving and muscles warm will help prevent any strains or injuries. Stretching after exercising is also important as it gives your muscles a chance to relax and stretch while they are warm. This also helps prevent injuries and cramps from happening.

Warm-Up Moves

CHEST OPENER

Time per rep: 10 seconds   **Total time: 1 minutes**

How to:

1. Stand up tall with feet hip-width distance apart. Hands are down by your sides.

2. Bring your hands behind you and clasp them together. Straighten both arms as you lift your hands slightly away from your buttocks and push out your chest.

3. Return hands down to the starting position.

4. Repeat five more times.

Take Note:

If you cannot clasp your hands behind you, it is okay. You can bring both hands behind you as you lift your arms as high as you can while pushing out your chest.

FORWARD FOLD

Time per rep: 15 seconds   **Total time: 1 minutes**

How to:

1. Stand up tall with feet hip-width distance apart. Hands are down by your sides.

2. Bring your hands behind you and clasp them together. Straighten both arms as you lift your hands slightly away from your buttocks and push out your chest.

3. Return hands down to the starting position.

4. Repeat five more times.

Take Note:

If you cannot clasp your hands behind you, it is okay. You can bring both hands behind you as you lift your arms as high as you can while pushing out your chest.

HIP CIRCLES

Time per rep: 15 seconds   **Total time: 1 minutes**

How to:

1. Stand with your feet hip-width distance apart, and knees slightly bent.

2. Place your hands on your hips.

3. Move your hips forward, right, back, and left. Repeat moving them in a clockwise motion for 30 seconds.

4. Switch directions and now move your hips counter-clockwise for another 30 seconds.

Take Note:

As you get warmed up, your hips will begin to move in a larger circle.

SIDE REACH

Time per rep: 15 seconds   **Total time: 1 minutes**

How to:

1. Stand erect with your feet hip-width distant apart. Hands are down by your sides.

2. Raise your right arm and bring your right hand over your head as you bend your torso to the left. Bring the arm down and return to the starting position.

3. Switch sides and raise your left arm up as you bend to the right. Return to the starting position.

4. Alternate bending right and then left for one minute.

Take Note:

Keep your chest facing straight in front of you as you bend from side to side

STANDING CAT COW

Time per rep: Varies   **Total time: 1 minutes**

How to:

1. Stand with your feet slightly wider than hip-width apart and knees bent.

2. Bend forward and place your hands on the tops of your knees.

3. Take a breath, inhaling as you drop your chin towards your chest and round your upper back (this is the cat position).

4. Exhale as you lift your chin to look up and arch your back, allowing your belly to relax towards your thighs (cow position).

5. Repeat the moves, alternating between cat and cow, for one minute.

Take Note:

Keep your shoulders relaxed throughout this warm-up exercise, and don't hunch up.

COOL DOWN STRETCHES
CAT COW

Time per rep: 10 seconds   **Total time: 1 minutes**

How to:

1. Get on your hands and knees on a mat on the floor. Hands are directly under your shoulders and knees directly under your hips.

2. Take a breath, inhaling as you drop your chin towards your chest and round your upper back (cat position).

3. Exhale as you lift your chin to look up and arch your back, allowing your belly to relax towards the floor (cow position).

4. Repeat the moves, alternating between cat and cow, for one minute.

Take Note:

Pay attention to any tightness in your upper and lower back. Adjust your stretch to accommodate your mobility in these areas.

CHILD'S POSE

Time per rep: 20 seconds   **Total time: 1 minutes**

How to:

1. Get on your hands and knees on a mat on the floor. Keeping your big toes together, widen your knees apart as far as comfortable.

2. Lower your hips to your feet while lowering your upper body and forehead down to the mat. Arms are out in front of you, reaching above your head, and hands are on the floor. Breathe in and out as you relax in this position for 10 seconds. Return to the starting position.

3. Repeat two more times.

Take Note:

If you have shoulder issues, it may be more comfortable for you to have your arms alongside your torso. Arms are resting on the floor with your palms facing up to the ceiling.

COBRA

Time per rep: 15 seconds   **Total time: 1 minutes**

How to:

1. Get on your hands and knees on a mat on the floor. Keeping your big toes together, widen your knees apart as far as comfortable.

2. Lower your hips to your feet while lowering your upper body and forehead down to the mat. Arms are out in front of you, reaching above your head, and hands are on the floor. Breathe in and out as you relax in this position for 10 seconds. Return to the starting position.

3. Repeat two more times.

Take Note:

It might be more comfortable for you to simply prop yourself up with your forearms on the floor rather than straightening your arms.

LEG CROSSOVER

Time per rep: 20 seconds   **Total time: 1 minutes**

How to:

1. Lie down with your back on the mat. Bend your knees, so they are pointing to-wards the ceiling. Bring your arms out into a T-position with your palms facing up.

2. Bring your right foot up and place it on top of your left knee. If needed, you can use your right hand to gently push your right knee away from you. Hold this position for five seconds.

3. Allow your left leg to slowly fall over to the left side and sole of your right foot to touch the floor, if possible. You might not be able to cross over all the way, and that's okay. Return to the starting position.

4. Switch legs. Place your left foot on your right knee. Let your right leg fall to the right, and your left sole to touch the floor. Return to starting positions and repeat once on each side.

Take Note:

Keep your chest facing up towards the ceiling at all times and the back of both shoulders firmly planted on the floor.

SEATED ROTATION

Time per rep: 15 seconds   **Total time: 1 minutes**

How to:

1. From a seated position, either in a chair or on the floor, sit up tall.

2. Cross your arms in front of you, keeping your shoulders relaxed.

3. Keeping your hips facing forward, turn your arms and upper torso to the right and look over your right shoulder. Hold this position for five seconds, then return to the starting position.

4. Now, turn your arms and torso to the left as you look over your left shoulder. Hold for five seconds, then return to the starting position.

5. Repeat the exercise once more on each side.

Take Note:

If you have had a neck injury or surgery, keep your head in line with your upper torso and don't look over your shoulder.

Walking Core Exercises

Walking is man's best medicine. —Hippocrates

Walking is a great way to get in some cardiovascular exercise, breathe in fresh air, and loosen muscles. It is a chance to get outdoors, enjoy the sunshine, and take in new views. Walking is also an opportunity to spend social time with others as you exercise together and build friendships. There are several core exercises that can be done while walking. While no equipment is needed, you can choose to add lightweight hand weights if you choose to.

ARM CURLS

Time per rep: 15 seconds   **Total time: 1 minutes**

How to:

1. Bend your arms at the elbows so that they form a 90-degree angle.
2. Slowly lower both hands down, then raise them up towards your shoulders. This is the same motion as doing a bicep curl.
3. Repeat the arm curls for one minute.

Level Up:

To make this more difficult, you can add one or two-pound weights in each hand.

Take Note:

Make this a slow and controlled movement. Don't pump your arms up and down.

LEG LIFT TOE TOUCHES

Time per rep: Varies   **Total time: 1 minutes**

How to:

1. Keeping it straight, lift your right leg as high as you can. At the same time, reach with your left hand towards your raised right foot as you twist your torso to the right. This requires some balance. Return to the starting position.
2. Switch legs. Lift your left leg and reach towards it with your opposite hand.
3. Continue to walk forward, lifting alternate legs, for one minute.

Level Up:

A variation of this is to lift just your knee instead of your entire leg.

Take Note:

Be sure you are walking on a level floor free from rocks and other things you could stumble over while doing this exercise.

PUNCH FORWARD

Time per rep: Varies   **Total time: 1 minutes**

How to:

1. Make a fist with both hands. Bring both hands up to the sides of your chest.

2. Punch your right fist out in front of you, slightly to the left of your torso and twisting your body slightly to the left. Bring your arm back.

3. Now, punch your left fist to the right of your torso and twist slightly to the right.

4. Repeat punching forward, alternating arms, for one minute.

Level Up:

You can make this more challenging by adding one or two-pound weights in each hand.

Take Note:

Be sure to tighten your abs and exhale as you punch each time.

SWING YOUR ARMS

Time per rep: Varies   **Total time: 1 minutes**

How to:

1. Bend your arms at the elbow, so they are at 90-degree angles.
2. As your right foot steps forward, swing your bent left arm forward.
3. When your left foot steps forward, swing your right arm forward.
4. Keep walking forward, swinging the opposite arm forward to help propel you along.

Level Up:

Adding one or two-pound weights in each hand will make this more difficult.

Take Note:

Ensure that whatever foot is forward, the opposite arm is forward. Having the same foot and arm forward at the same time will result in an awkward gait.

TIGHTEN YOUR TUMMY

Time per rep: Varies   **Total time: 1 minutes**

How to:

1. As you walk, draw in your abdominal muscles and lift your chest.

2. Keep these muscles engaged for one minute or as long as you can.

3. Repeat the exercise a few times during your walk.

Level Up:

You can place your hand on your belly as a reminder to keep your core engaged as you walk.

Take Note:

Keep your shoulders relaxed and maintain good posture as you tighten your core muscles.

WALK UPHILL

Time per rep: Varies   **Total time: 1 minutes**

How to:

1. Find a walking path that includes an incline or uphill section.

2. As you walk up the incline, swing your arms to help propel you up the hill. Engage your buttock muscles and tighten your abdominals as you trek the incline.

Level Up:

Incorporating an incline into your walks several times a week will make your walks more challenging.

Take Note:

Don't lean your chest too far forward as you walk uphill. Maintain good posture and a relaxed neck and upper back.

Weekly
Schedules

The secret of your future is hidden in your daily routine. —Mike Murdock

It is time to put all you have learned into an action plan! In this chapter, you will find weekly schedules that incorporate the core exercises into easy-to-follow plans.

There are three weeks of routines, six days per week. This leaves room for rest days and for the unexpected day off. Many people believe that twenty-one days of doing something builds a new habit. In reality, it takes longer than that, but three weeks is a good kick-start towards your goal of a stronger core and improved stability as you age.

- ○ Five days start with a warm-up exercise, include three core exercises, and end with a cool down exercise.

- ○ There is a daily focus of either mat, seated, or standing moves.

- ○ One day is devoted to walking and the core exercises that accompany it.

- ○ If you have a partner available, you can do the partner exercise as well.

WEEK 1 SCHEDULE

Day 1

- ○ Warm-up: Side Reach
- ○ Mat Core Exercises: Dead Bug, Mountain Climber, Superman
- ○ Partner Exercise: Partner Reach and Touch Plank
- ○ Cool down: Child's Pose

Day 2

- ○ Warm-up: Chest Opener
- ○ Seated Core Exercises: Seated Side Bend, Forward Roll Up, Seated Leg Lift
- ○ Partner Exercise: Partner Russian Twist and Pass
- ○ Cool down: Cobra

Day 3

- ○ Warm-up: Forward Fold
- ○ Standing Core Exercises: Standing Bird Dog, Figure 8 Row, Squat
- ○ Partner Exercise: Partner Squat with Both Hands
- ○ Cool down: Cat Cow

Day 4

- ○ Warm-up: Hip Circles
- ○ Mat Core Exercises: Modified Curl Up, Segment Rotation, Plank
- ○ Partner Exercise: Partner Leg Raise Push Down
- ○ Cool down: Seated Rotation

Day 5

- ○ Warm-up: Standing Cat Cow
- ○ Seated Core Exercises: Seated Twist, Half Roll Back, Single Knee Tuck
- ○ Partner Exercise: Partner Heel Tap
- ○ Cool down: Leg Crossover Stretch

Day 6 - Walk

- ○ Warm-up: Side Reach
- ○ Walking Exercises: Swing Your Arms, Walk Uphill
- ○ Cool down: Child's Pose

Day 1

- ○ Warm-up: Chest Opener
- ○ Standing Core Exercises: Standing Side Bend, Core Rotation, Knee Rotation
- ○ Partner Exercise: Partner Push
- ○ Cool down: Cobra

Day 2

- ○ Warm-up: Forward Fold
- ○ Mat Core Exercises: Bridge, Side Plank, Single Leg Abdominal Press
- ○ Partner Exercise: Partner Get Ups
- ○ Cool down: Cat Cow

Day 3

- ○ Warm-up: Hip Circles
- ○ Seated Core Exercises: Seated Dead Bug, Leg Taps, Seated Russian Twist
- ○ Partner Exercise: Partner Hand Shadows
- ○ Cool down: Leg Crossover Stretch

Day 4

- ○ Warm-up: Standing Cat Cow
- ○ Standing Core Exercises: Standing Twist, Standing Bicycle Crunch, Wide Side Crunch
- ○ Partner Exercise: Partner Squat with Both Hands
- ○ Cool down: Seated Rotation

Day 5

- ○ Warm-up: Side Reach
- ○ Mat Core Exercises: Bird Dog, Side Plank with Rotation, Supine Toe Tap
- ○ Partner Exercise: Partner Reach and Touch Plank
- ○ Cool down: Child's Pose

Day 6 - Walk

- ○ Warm-up: Chest Opener
- ○ Walking Exercises: Punch Forward, Tighten Your Tummy
- ○ Cool down: Cobra

Day 1

- ○ Warm-up: Forward Fold
- ○ Seated Core Exercises: Band Extension, Resisted Knee Lift, Seated Jumping Jack
- ○ Partner Exercise: Partner Heel Tap
- ○ Cool down: Leg Crossover Stretch

Day 2

- ○ Warm-up: Hip Circles
- ○ Standing Core Exercises: Standing Crunch, Knee Tuck Extension, Woodchops
- ○ Partner Exercise: Partner Hand Shadow
- ○ Cool down: Seated Rotation

Day 3

- ○ Warm-up: Standing Cat Cow
- ○ Mat Core Exercises: Dead Bug, Mountain Climber, Superman
- ○ Partner Exercise: Partner Russian Twist and Pass
- ○ Cool down: Cat Cow

Day 4

- ○ Warm-up: Side Reach
- ○ Seated Core Exercises: Seated Side Bend, Forward Roll-Up, Seated Leg Lift
- ○ Partner Exercise: Partner Leg Raise Push Down
- ○ Cool down: Child's Pose

Day 5

- ○ Warm-up: Chest Opener
- ○ Standing Core Exercises: Standing Bird Dog, Figure 8 Row, Squat
- ○ Partner Exercise: Partner Get Up
- ○ Cool down: Cobra

Day 6 - Walk

- ○ Warm-up: Forward Fold
- ○ Walking Exercises: Arm Curls, Leg Lift Toe Touches
- ○ Cool down: Leg Crossover Stretch

Conclusion

You made it! Congratulations on taking charge of your health and well-being by choosing to learn how to age well. As we have traveled this journey together, we have discovered a lot about our bodies and how they function. So, many factors contribute to how our bodies respond to the number of years we live on this earth. Some elements we cannot control, but those that we can include diet, exercise, and the choices we make.

One of the pillars of aging well is having a core of strength and flexibility. Because our core muscles are responsible for our ability to accomplish everyday tasks, engage in physical activities, and even play with our grandchildren. They play an essential role in our overall vitality. Early on in the book, we looked at the disadvantages of having a weak core versus the advantages of maintaining a strong one. Then, we assessed the state of our core strengths and weaknesses with a simple quiz.

The following chapters outlined a variety of core exercises that can immediately be put into practice. The core exercises we learned comprised of:

- Mat core exercises. These twelve exercises are done close to the floor on all fours or lying down and help us increase our ability to get up and down more easily.

- Seated core exercises. Able to be done by those who have trouble standing or getting on the floor, these twelve exercises helped us build our core strength from a seated position.

- Standing core exercises. Balance and stability are significant components in core strength and working through the twelve standing exercises helped train our muscles for everyday activities.

- Partner core exercises. These eight exercises added a little fun and encouragement as we worked on our core with a workout partner.

- Warm-up and cool down. Often overlooked, these warm-ups and cool down stretches help our muscles transition from inactivity to activity and back.

- Walking core exercises. Doing double duty, these exercises work the core muscles and can be done while getting in a walk.

Finally, we looked at incorporating all that we have learned into a weekly workout schedule. Depending on your preferences and goals, you can work through each exercise at your own pace, doing one a day, until you work through all fifty exercises. For those looking for a ready-made plan, the daily routines listed provide an easy way to complete the exercises in this book without having to come up with your plan.

My hope and desire is that you will benefit from the information and encouragement in this book. If you found this book helpful, please consider leaving a review and letting me know your thoughts! I look forward to hearing how implementing these exercises into your daily plan of exercise and wellness helps you build strength and stability in your core.

Scan The QR Code to Leave a Review:

I hope you enjoy good health and happiness on the long road ahead of you, and I wish you all the best. Thank you for allowing me to share my knowledge with you.

-Baz Thompson

Stretching Exercises for Seniors

Simple Movements to Improve Posture, Decrease Back Pain, and Prevent Injury After 60

Baz Thompson

Introduction

Stretching is an activity you may think you don't need to do. You might say, "I'm not a gymnast or a football player. Why would I need to stretch?" While athletes of all kinds do practice stretching as part of their quest to maintain their competitive edge, all types of folks also stretch to benefit their bodies and general well-being. Regular stretching helps keep our muscles strong and pliable. This helps with flexibility in our muscles, ligaments, tendons, and joints (Harvard Health Publishing, 2013). By sustaining our flexibility, we keep our full range of motion, which allows us to continue the activities we enjoy.

Our normal range of activities that we do every day contributes to our need for stretching. When we stay seated for any length of time, the muscles in the back of our legs become tight. This makes it difficult to straighten our legs all the way, resulting in an increase in pain when we walk. Something as simple as walking can become harder to do when our muscles are tight and joints are stiff. When we ask our tight muscles to suddenly spring into action, for something fun like dancing with our partner or for something imperative like jumping out of the way of an oncoming bicycle, they may pull or tear because of the strain. Muscles that are not strong enough to support us in everyday tasks can lead to falls and other serious injuries.

Regular stretching keeps our muscles from contraction and stiffness. By keeping them elongated, flexible, and healthy, we protect our joints, ligaments, and tendons as well. It is not necessary to stretch all our muscles every day. Doctors and physical therapists like David Nolan of Massachusetts General Hospital recommend concentrating most stretches on the major muscle groups that affect our mobility (Harvard Health Publishing, 2013). This includes lower body muscles such as hip flexors, hamstrings (back of thigh), quadriceps (front of thigh), and calves. Also recommended are upper body stretches that target areas of tension like the neck, shoulders, and lower back.

We've all heard the saying that Rome was not built in a day, and the same can be said for flexibility. Stretching a few times will not make you less stiff and more flexible. The effects of stretching are cumulative, meaning that they build over time. Just as your stiffness and immobility did not happen overnight, the looseness and limberness of your muscles will not happen right away. It can take months to become more flexible and it takes regular stretching to maintain it. The result is strong, supple muscles that are flexible and supportive of joints and connective tissue. This contributes to our quality of life, especially as we age.

This book looks at stretching as a way to maintain good posture, decrease back pain, and help prevent injury as we progress past the age of sixty. The older population can especially benefit from a regular stretching routine. Getting older can sometimes mean a decrease in strenuous activity, an increase in surgeries, and less mobility because of disease or age. While stretching can't fix everything, it can bring movement and increased flexibility back to a person's life in their older years. In the first chapter, we will look at what happens to our bodies as we get older and the particular benefits that come from regular stretching. We will also learn about the types of stretching and when, where, and how to do it. The following chapters are dedicated to the times of day to stretch such as morning, evening, pre-activity, and post-activity. Included are the explanations and illustrations of each stretch and what areas of the body they benefit. Lastly, there is a chapter on target area stretches that focus on the smaller muscles of the body that profit from stretching.

As always, check with your doctor or healthcare provider before starting on any exercise or stretching regimen particularly if you have had a recent injury, are recovering from surgery, or have a chronic health condition.

Are you ready? Let's get your fitness education and training started!

The Power of Stretching

Stretching is good for our bodies at any age, but in this chapter, we will examine why it is especially important to stretch as we get older. We will take a look at what happens physiologically to our bodies as we progress in years, including what things we can do to prevent ourselves from further problems and injury. Next, we will talk about the benefits of stretching and why even a little bit of daily stretching will keep us from pain and stiffness. We will learn about the types of stretches we can do that are beneficial, plus highlight what kinds of stretches to avoid. Finally, we will talk about when, where, and how to stretch for everyone from beginner to experienced stretchers.

OUR BODIES AS WE AGE

In the past, the older population was lumped together in one large group known as the elderly. With average life spans increasing, however, older adults are now subdivided into smaller age range groups. The adult population over 65 can be divided into three groups:

- Young Old (ages 65 to 74).
- Middle Old (ages 75 to 84).
- Old Old (ages 85 and older).

Someone who is 65 years old will have very different muscle strength, cognitive awareness, physical abilities, and injury recovery time than someone who is 90 years old. In one study, it was found that those in the Young Old group had lower hospital admission rates and quicker hospital discharge rates than those in the Old Old group (Lee, et al., 2018). It is important to note that our chronological age, the actual number of years we have lived on earth, is only one way to measure our age. There is also our biological age to consider.

Biological age refers to our level of physical fitness, mental acuity, and overall health. We can see this when we compare two people who are the same chronological age but who differ greatly in their biological age. One person who is 70 years old may have arthritis, limited mobility in their hands and knees, constant brain fog, and consume a diet high in processed foods and sugar. The other 70 year old person may have diabetes but still have the ability to play tennis twice a week, practice yoga daily, complete crossword puzzles regularly, and eat lots of fresh vegetables and fruits. Chronological age is something we don't have control over, but our biological age is one that we exert some control by the choices we make.

Our level of physical and mental fitness, or biological age, has several contributing factors. One factor is the DNA that we are born with in our cells. Some people are born with a propensity for disease or frailty that is determined by their inherited genes. Obviously, this factor cannot be changed, regardless of what we do. There are other factors, however, that are in our control. These factors include healthy food choices; regular exercise and stretching; maintenance of mental sharpness, emotional balance, and social connections.

We know that as the years pass, we get older and our bodies change. With the advancement of medical technology and preventative medicine, humans are able to live longer and have a better quality of life than our ancestors. However, we cannot stop the natural decline of certain faculties and the damage that happens to our cells with the passage of time. When we are young, our cells have the ability to repair themselves quickly and with minimal draw from energy resources in the body (National Center for Biotechnology Information, U.S. Library of Medicine, 2020). As we get older, the cells do not turn over as quickly and that slow down in cell turnover adds up, eventually resulting in signs of aging.

Our bodies are composed of many different types of cells. Some cells are short-lived, so they are constantly being replaced by new ones. An example of this type of cell is our skin cells. As we grow older, this replacement doesn't happen as quickly. With skin cells, this slow down in replacement cells can be seen in the form of skin wrinkles, less elasticity, and dryness. Other cells are long-lived, but when they die they are never replaced. Cells in the brain are an example of this type.

Muscle cells, even in older adults, are self-renewing. One of the natural consequences of growing older is a loss of muscle mass and strength which contributes to frailty and immobility. This often results in falls and an increased risk for injury. Certain lifestyle choices, however, can help slow down the loss of muscle. According to a recent study (McCormick & Vasilaki, 2018), these factors include:

- Increase in protein consumption.
- Aerobic exercise.
- Resistance training.
- Other forms of physical activity like stretching.

Paying attention to these factors and choosing to apply them in our lives helps slow the loss of muscle mass and muscle strength as we grow older. Some researchers have concluded that "...Exercise training and proper nutrition can have dramatic effects on muscle mass and strength" (Volpi, et al., 2004).

The Benefits of Stretching

When it is done correctly, stretching feels good. The American Council on Exercise says that flexibility is an essential part of fitness and should be incorporated into a regular workout program (American Council on Exercise, 2014). They list 10 benefits of stretching, including:

- Increased blood flow to muscles and joints, plus increased circulation of blood throughout the body.
- Loosening of muscles in preparation for exercise.
- Relieves post-exercise aches and pains.
- Improves range of motion and decreases muscle stiffness.
- Decreases resistance of muscles, leading to possible decrease in injury.
- Improves posture and alignment of shoulder, spine, and hip muscles.

- Allows muscle relaxation and reduces muscle tension.
- Reduces lower back pain.
- Creates more efficient joint movement which makes movements require less energy.
- Reduces overall stress in the body.

In a study done on women between the ages of 62 and 74, researchers looked specifically at the knee flexors of the women in the study. After three months of participating in an active stretching program, the women were found to have increased flexibility and torque (twisting ability) in their knee flexors, which are the muscles that surround and decrease the angle of the knees, such as the hamstrings (Batista, et al., 2009). This increase in flexibility provided more functional mobility in all the women.

THE TYPES OF STRETCHING

When we think of stretching, we may remember how we used to stretch when we were in an elementary school physical education class. Do you remember standing and bending over, trying to touch your feet while bouncing from the waist? Or sitting on the floor, legs apart, and trying to touch your toes while stretching and bouncing? This type of stretching is known as ballistic stretching. The premise of ballistic stretching uses force, gravity, or momentum to stretch your muscle past its normal range of motion by repeatedly bouncing or pushing. While this mode of stretching has fallen out of favor because of the increased possibility of muscle tears and pulls, some professional athletes and dancers still use it. This type of stretching is not recommended for most people, and especially not for older adults.

Popular in today's medical and fitness worlds are dynamic stretching and static stretching. What is the difference between the two? Dynamic stretching is used prior to exercising, team sports, or any strenuous activity. The purpose of dynamic stretching is to get the muscles ready that you will be using in the activity by increasing the temperature of the muscles and decreasing any muscle stiffness. These stretches take your muscles and joints through the range of motion slowly before you perform them with more intensity and speed. Examples of dynamic stretches are walking lunges, torso twists, arm circles, and leg swings. Many dynamic stretches are sport specific, meaning they mimic the movement you will be doing in your particular sport or workout.

Static stretching is used after exercise to help you cool down and stretch out muscles, but it is also used as part of a routine stretching program to help maintain flexibility and mobility in your muscles and joints. Stretching a muscle as far as it can go without pain and holding the stretch for 30 to 60 seconds is the basic idea of static stretching. Holding a stretched position helps lengthen your muscles, increasing flexibility, and helps relax your muscles. Examples of static stretches are hamstring stretch, side bends, and hip flexor stretch. Static stretches are done standing, sitting, or lying down.

WHEN, WHERE, AND HOW TO STRETCH

In this section, we will look at the basics of stretching and learn when, where, and how to stretch.

WHEN TO STRETCH

We have already touched on the importance of stretching before exercising or activity and afterwards. The pre-activity stretches are meant to warm up muscles for an increase in muscular activity through exercise, dance, or other sport. These stretches don't help with flexibility but are preparation for increased movement. Post-activity stretches are done while you are cooling down from an exercise or activity. Your muscles are easier to stretch because they are warm and supple, making them more flexible. But what about other times of the day that stretching can be done?

Stretching in the morning just after waking up is a great way to release tension and to help you gently wake up your body. The body heals and does repair work on itself while you are sleeping and that includes repair of muscles and other soft tissue (Walker, 2010). When you awaken in the morning, increasing your circulation flow brings blood and oxygen into your muscles at a higher rate and gets your body ready for the events of the day ahead. Morning stretches also help wake up your joints and alleviate any stiffness from them being still and immobile most of the night.

A short stretch break done several times during the day is helpful to keep joints and muscles loose and moving. If you do a lot of sitting for work or in your leisure time, it's important to get up and stretch your neck, upper back, lower back, and hips to keep them limber. Stretch breaks are also great ways to take a mental break from whatever work or activity you are doing. By concentrating on your body and the movements it is making as you stretch, along with some focused breathing, you can come back to your work relaxed and renewed.

Most people do not think of stretching in the evening before going to bed, but this is a great time to stretch! As we discussed earlier, your muscles and soft tissues like ligaments and tendons are repaired while you sleep. By stretching in the evening, you elongate and lengthen your muscles. This increased muscle length allows the repair and healing work to be done along the entire muscle (Walker, 2010). Also, stretching before bedtime is a way to wind down and relax. The slow, rhythmic movements of a gentle stretching routine, along with measured breathing, help signal the body and mind that sleep is coming.

WHERE TO STRETCH

The best place to stretch is anywhere that you have enough room and are comfortable. This could be in your bedroom, living room, home gym, backyard, or garage. It is also possible to stretch outdoors at a park, beach, or open air sports facility. The important thing is to check the surroundings to be sure that you are stretching on a level surface to avoid any imbalances or falls. Having a padded exercise or yoga mat can be helpful, especially if you are doing stretches that involve kneeling, sitting, or lying on the ground. Seated stretches can be done from a chair at your desk, dining room table, or even in your car.

HOW TO STRETCH

Stretching requires more than just bending over and reaching for your toes. Proper form such as breathing, variety, and alignment all contribute to getting the most out of your stretching routine. Being aware of common mistakes and avoiding them is also important.

Breathing seems like a natural thing to do. We all do it several thousand times a day. Proper breathing allows for full expansion of your entire lungs. Many people breathe by taking shallow breaths that cause their chest to rise and fall and their waist to contract and get small. These types of breaths miss filling the lower part of your lungs. The proper way to breathe, sometimes called belly breathing, is to breathe into your belly and diaphragm area. To do this, sit or lie down comfortably and breathe in through your nose. Your chest and belly should expand, and then exhale through your mouth. Belly breathing takes some practice, but gets easier as you practice it more.

Doing some stretching every day is a good idea, especially if you are working on flexibility or recovery of a particular muscle. Just as you wouldn't eat the same thing everyday or do the same exercise day in and day out, you also don't want to do the same stretches all the time. Including several different types of stretches is important to avoid any muscle imbalances or overworking of muscles.

Good posture and body alignment are important to avoid strain and injury, and that goes for stretching, too. Maintaining proper posture and good form as you stretch helps ensure that the muscles you are targeting are being stretched properly and that you are not putting unnecessary pressure on your neck or other joints. There is a tendency for some people to scrunch their shoulders or hunch over while stretching. This causes imbalance and undue tension on those areas that may lead to injury. Maintain good posture and alignment by keeping your back straight (but not rigid), shoulders down and away from your ears, and your jaw relaxed.

According to the Stretch Coach, author and stretching guru Brad Walker, there are some common mistakes that people make when they start out stretching (Walker, 2010). These include:

- ○ Holding your breath. This causes muscles to tense up and become difficult to stretch. Breathe deeply using the belly breathing technique to relax muscles and increase circulation.

- ○ Forgetting to warm up. Walker likens this to stretching old, dry rubber bands. They don't stretch very far and may snap. Take five minutes to warm up your muscles by walking in place to increase muscle temperature and make them more pliable.

- ○ Stretching an injury. If injured, there should not be any stretching done for the first 72 hours. For the first two weeks, very gentle and light static stretching can be done. After that some dynamic stretching can slowly be reintroduced into your stretching routine.

- ○ Stretching to the point of pain. When we stretch too hard, our muscles employ a built-in safety reflex. They naturally contract to get away and protect the body from the pain. Stretch only to where it is comfortable and a slight tension.

- ○ Not holding the stretch long enough. Holding the position for just a few seconds may feel like a stretch, but it isn't long enough for the muscle to relax and lengthen. It is important to hold a stretch position for 30 to 60 seconds, about two or three deep breaths, and repeat the stretch two or three more times.

Stretching is beneficial to our bodies and especially so as we grow older. However, it is not a quick fix. It will take time to see the results of a regular stretching routine, but the benefits to your body and well being are worth it!

Morning
Stretches

A morning stretch after a night's rest is not only a good way to wake up, but it also is a way to relax muscles that have been stagnant and still all night. When we sleep, our heart rate slows down, muscles relax, and blood flow slows down. It is a time when our body can rest and rejuvenate. That is why it is common when waking up for our body to be stiff because of muscle inactivity while resting. This is especially true if you sleep in the same position all night. Also, while we sleep, the fluid increases in our joints and spine and can lead to extra stiffness and morning aches (Stretch22, n.d.). As we get older this stiffness, when combined with arthritis or other health challenges, can be somewhat painful and can linger throughout the morning. Stretching helps alleviate this stiffness and joint discomfort. It also gets the body moving and ready for the day ahead. By stretching in the morning on a regular basis, you are increasing the mobility of your muscles and joints. The increased mobility and flexibility helps prevent future injury.

Remember that morning stretches are your body's chance to awaken, increase the blood flow, and get the muscles warmed up. Because muscles can be very tight in the morning, your range of flexibility is less than it would be later in the day. You will not be able to stretch as far or as deep as you normally would, but that is perfectly okay. Be especially careful not to do any bouncing or bobbing while doing the stretches as this can cause pulled or torn muscles. It is important to be kind to your body, especially so early in the day. Stretching in the morning should feel good!

Most of the upper body stretches can be done standing or sitting, so choose what is most appropriate for you. Doing the stretches while standing helps energize your body in the morning, but if you can't stand for any period of time it is fine to sit while performing the stretches. The lower body stretches are done on the floor, but use a padded mat if it is more comfortable for you. A padded mat is important if you have any knee pain or hip issues. Since these are stretches that are done in the morning, you can do these stretches in your bedroom, if you have the space. Almost all of the stretches, with the exception of a few lower body stretches, can even be done in your pajamas while still in bed! Use common sense and precautions to be sure your bed and surroundings are safe to perform any stretching exercises before starting.

You do not have to do all the stretches in this chapter every morning unless you want to. If pressed for time, choose one upper body and one lower body stretch and do just those. Even stretching for five minutes is a helpful start to your day.

Upper Body Stretches

OVERHEAD STRETCH

Areas stretched: chest, shoulders, triceps, lats, front of neck.

1. Standing with feet about hips width apart, raise both arms above your head.

2. Reach fingers, hands, and arms up as if you are trying to touch the ceiling. Take a deep breath in and then exhale.

3. If comfortable, look up and point your chin straight in front of you. Deep breath and exhale. If you have any neck pain or neck issues, skip this step.

4. With hands still raised, slightly bend the upper body backwards and hold for 2 or 3 seconds, then return to standing straight.

5. Lower arms back down to sides.

6. Repeat the stretch two or three times.

Take note:

This can be done seated if you are unsteady on your feet or if you have any vertigo or balance issues.

CACTUS ARMS

Areas stretched: front of the shoulder, chest.

1. From a standing or seated position, raise arms overhead and then lower to bend at the elbow to form 90 degree angles, palms facing forward. Your arms should form a cactus or football goal post shape.

2. With arms still raised and bent, push your chest forward as you push your arms slightly backward. Take a deep breath, then exhale and bring your chest and arms back to normal.

3. Repeat two or three times.

Take note:

Protect your lower back if you are standing or sitting by not arching your lower back while doing this stretch. If you find you are arching, you can do this stretch lying on your back and taking care to keep your lower back pressed to the floor.

NECK ROLL STRETCH

Areas stretched: back and sides of neck, trapezius.

1. From a standing or seated position, look straight ahead. Slowly tilt your head to the left as if your left ear was trying to touch the top of your left shoulder. Be sure your shoulders do not hunch up! Keep them relaxed and down. Take a deep breath in and then exhale.

2. Slowly roll your head down so that your chin is pointing towards your chest. Remember to keep the shoulders relaxed. Deep breath in and then exhale.

3. Roll your head to the right. Your right ear should be facing down as if to touch the top of your right shoulder. Deep breath in and then exhale. Slowly bring the head back to a neutral upright position. You can use your hands to gently help your head come back to upright.

4. Repeat two or three times. You can alternate sides by starting with the right side first.

Take note:

Never tilt your head back while doing neck rolls. This puts a lot of unnecessary compression on your neck and spine.

SEATED SPINAL TWIST

Areas stretched: entire back, upper glutes.

1. Sitting on the floor cross legged, sit up tall and gently twist your upper body to the right. Place your left hand on your right knee and your right hand on the floor behind you.

2. If you can, look to the back over your right shoulder. If not, keep your head relaxed and look ahead or down. Take a deep breath in, then exhale.

3. Return your upper body and head back to the front. Take a deep breath in, then exhale.

4. Change the cross of your legs, now putting the other leg in front.

5. Sit up tall and gently twist your upper body to the left. Place your right hand on your left knee and your left hand on the floor behind you.

6. Look to the back over your left shoulder, if possible. Otherwise, relax your neck and look ahead or down. Take a deep breath in, and then exhale.

7. Return your upper body and head back to the front. Repeat the stretch two or three more times.

Take note:

Keep both glutes firmly on the ground. If one side is lifting up, you are twisting too far. Only twist as far as you are comfortable.

CAT AND COW

Areas stretched: upper back, mid back, back of neck, shoulders.

1. Get on your hands and knees on the floor. Your hands should be directly under your shoulders and your knees directly under your hips. Your back should be neutral and roughly parallel to the floor.

2. Take a deep breath and inhale while gently lifting your head and your tailbone. Your back will arch slightly and your belly will hang and be loose. This is called the cow stretch.

3. While exhaling, gently lower your chin towards your chest as you round your upper back towards the ceiling. Keep your tailbone and your abdominals tucked in but don't clench them. This portion is called the cat stretch.

4. Repeat the cow and cat stretches slowly, flowing from one to the other, several times.

Take note:

Keep your shoulders away from your ears and relaxed while doing this stretch. There should not be any tension in your neck or shoulders.
If your wrists cannot support you, a variation of this stretch can be done seated. Sit cross legged and place your hands on your knees while doing the cat and cow stretches.

Lower Body Stretches

EATED FORWARD BEND

Areas stretched: Entire back of body including calves, hamstrings, and back.

1. Sit on the floor with your legs together and straight out in front of you. Legs can be slightly apart.

2. Raise both arms overhead with palms facing each other. Take a deep breath in and then exhale.

3. While exhaling, bend your upper body forward from the hip joint. Keep your neck in a neutral position and your back straight. It is okay to have a slight bend at your knees; they don't have to be perfectly straight

4. Bring your arms down and let hands rest on the floor with palms facing up.

5. Repeat the stretch by raising arms overhead and starting again. Do this two or three more times.

Take note:

Remember not to bounce when folding forward and don't force yourself to try to go lower. Hamstrings and calves are naturally tight in the morning. This should be a fairly passive stretch that just loosens up the back of the legs and back.

FOOT POINT AND FLEX

Areas stretched: toes, feet, ankles, calves.

1. In a seated position on the floor with your legs straight out in front of you, point the feet and toes. Stretch them as far away from you as you can. Take a deep breath in and then exhale.

2. In the same seated position, flex your feet and toes back so that toes point up to the ceiling and maybe even flex towards you. Take a deep breath in and then exhale.

3. Repeat the stretch two or three more times.

Take note:

This stretch can be done seated in a chair if the floor is too uncomfortable. You can also stretch one foot at a time if you find it too hard to do both feet at the same time.

HALF KNEELING HIP FLEXOR STRETCH

Areas stretched: hip flexor, quads.

1. Start on the floor by coming down on all fours with both hands and both knees on the ground. Get into a half kneeling position by lifting the left knee and bringing the left foot forward in front of you. Left foot should be directly under the left knee.

2. Raise up so that your body is upright and your right knee is on the ground directly below your right hip. Both knees should be at a 90 degree angle and hands on your hips. Take a deep breath in and exhale.

3. While exhaling, move hips forward. Your weight will transfer to your left foot and you will feel the front of your right hip stretch. Keep an upright posture. Take a deep breath in and then exhale. Move hips back to starting position.

4. Repeat the stretch two or three more times on the same leg. Switch legs to stretch your other hip flexor.

Take note:

Hip flexors are tight in most people and that contributes to back pain. Take this stretch slowly and allow your hip flexor to relax. As you do this stretch more regularly, you will be able to come forward farther.

If you are stable and confident in this stretch, you can make it more challenging by lifting your arms above your head while stretching.

LYING KNEES TO CHEST

Areas stretched: lower back, hips, glutes, hamstrings.

1. Lie down on your back, resting your legs and arms on the floor.

2. Bring your left knee up towards your chest and place your hands either on top or behind your knee to support your leg. Don't tug or pull on your leg. Take a deep breath in and then exhale. Return your leg to the starting position.

3. Draw your right knee up towards your chest and either place your hands on top of the knee or behind it. Remember not to pull on your leg. Take a deep breath in and then exhale. Return your leg back down to the floor.

4. Repeat the sequence two or three more times.

Take note:

Once you are comfortable and confident in this stretch, you can make it more challenging by drawing up both knees at the same time. Either place hands on top of knees or one hand behind each knee for support.

ALL FOURS SIDE BEND

Areas stretched: sides of hips, torso, and neck.

1. Get on all fours on the floor with hands directly below shoulders and knees directly below hips.

2. Pick up the left leg and bring it over the right leg and foot. Place the left foot on the floor as far to the right as you can comfortably get it.

3. Look over the right shoulder and back at your foot. Take a deep breath, lean into your left hip, and then exhale. You should feel the stretch along the entire left side of your body.

4. Bring the left leg back to the starting position. Breathe in and out.

5. Now, pick up the right leg and take it over the other leg and foot. Place the right foot on the floor as far to the left as you can.

6. Look over the left shoulder and back at your foot. Take a deep breath, lean into your right hip this time, and then exhale. Feel the stretch along the right side of your body. Bring legs back to the starting position.

7. Repeat the stretch on both legs two more times.

Take note:

This is a deep stretch along the sides of the body and should feel good, especially in the morning. If you have neck issues, you don't have to look over your shoulder if it causes any pain. You can just concentrate on stretching the lower body.

Evening and Bedtime Stretch- es

Stretching in the evening and just before bedtime is a wonderful way to wind down. Many people have a difficult time falling asleep at night. Sometimes the inability to relax before bedtime is related to our muscles feeling restless. If you have had a day of sitting in a chair at work, sitting in a car, or just sitting at home, your muscles need some movement and stretching to release the tension that has built up during the day. Along with releasing tension, stretching also increases circulation and blood flow to tense muscles (Sleep Advisor, 2020). Once the muscles have been stretched and relaxed, you will be less likely to toss and turn once you get into bed to go to sleep. This increase in the quality of your sleep is not only a benefit to you, but also to your partner who may awaken when you sleep restlessly.

When you relax the body, it's natural for your mind to also relax and get ready for sleep. By doing a regular night time stretching routine, your mind and body know it is the time that they can enter into a calming, loosening, and relaxing state. This focused state of deliberately relaxing helps you to separate the activity phase of your day from the restful phase of your night. Slow and deliberate breathing while performing these stretches also contributes to entering into a relaxed state. If you find that you are inadvertently holding your breath while stretching, you may be stretching too intensely or too fast. Your goal is to deepen and slow your breathing. Relaxing your body and your mind allows you to release the stress and tension of the day and leave it behind. This release may help you fall asleep faster and stay asleep longer.

If desired, you can take a warm bath or shower prior to performing these stretching exercises. This helps wash off your day both mentally and physically. It also adds a marker to your evening routine that signals to both body and mind that sleep is coming. Performing the evening stretches after a warm shower also warms up the muscles prior to stretching. Most of the evening stretches are done low to the ground and can even be done in bed, if you choose. If the stretches are done on the floor, do them on a padded mat or on your bedroom carpet. As always, look at your bed and surroundings to be sure they are safe to perform these stretching exercises on and use common sense.

Remember, you do not have to do every stretch in this chapter every evening. The goal is to unwind and loosen up, so choose one upper body stretch and one lower body stretch to do in the evening. Taking just five minutes to stretch before bedtime will help you relax before drifting off to sleep.

Upper Body Stretches

BEAR HUG

Areas stretched: upper and middle back including trapezius and shoulder blades.

1. From a standing or seated position, raise both arms out from the sides of your body, palms facing forward. Take a deep breath in and then exhale.

2. Take another deep breath in and gently cross your arms in front of you, right arm over left. Exhaling, give yourself a hug. Your hands should be touching the back of your shoulders. Hold this position and breathe in and out slowly two more times.

3. Release your arms and bring them back to your sides.

4. Breathing deep, gently cross your arms again, this time with your left arm over your right. Exhale and hug yourself. You may be able to bring your hands onto your shoulder blades, but if not just keep them on your shoulders. Hold this position and slowly breathe in and out two more times.

5. Release your arms. Repeat if you desire or move on to another stretch.

Take note:

Depending on the length of your arms and the size of your chest, you may or may not be able to touch your shoulder blades. The goal here is to stretch the muscles of your upper back.

Remember to not scrunch up your shoulders. Keep them down and away from your ears.

SEATED OVERHEAD SIDE STRETCH

Areas stretched: entire sides of the body, neck, upper arms.

1. From a seated position, sitting cross legged, raise your left arm above your head and reach for the ceiling. Take a deep breath in.

2. As you exhale, bend your head and torso to the right while looking straight ahead. If it is okay for you, let your neck relax and allow your head to also bend to the right. You can place the other hand on the floor for balance. Take a slow, deep breath in and then exhale. Breathe in and out a couple of more times before returning to the starting position.

3. Change the cross of your legs. Raise your right arm up and reach for the ceiling. Take a deep breath in.

4. Exhaling, bend your head and torso to the left while keeping your gaze straight ahead. If possible, let your neck relax and let your head also bend to the left. Place your other hand on the floor for balance if you need to. Slowly breathe in and then exhale. Breathe in and out a few more times and then return to the starting position.

Take note:

Don't allow your chest to fall forward or your shoulders to round during this stretch. Maintain good posture while doing this stretch by engaging your abdominal core muscles. Be sure to keep both glutes firmly on the floor. If one or the other is lifting up as you stretch to the side, you are stretching too far.

THREAD THE NEEDLE

Areas stretched: shoulders, upper arms, neck, spine.

1. Get on the floor on all fours. Hands should be directly under your shoulders and knees directly under your hips.

2. Take your left hand and thread it under your right arm and just above the floor. Continue extending your left arm along the floor as you bring your left shoulder to the floor. Let your left hand rest on the floor, palm facing up. Your left ear should be resting on the floor as well.

3. Slide the other hand along the floor until it is above your head, palm down, so it is touching the floor just past your head. If this is too much, just leave your right hand where it is. Take a deep, slow breath in and then exhale. Your neck should be relaxed. Breathe slowly in and out two more times. Slowly lift your shoulder up and return to starting position.

4. To do the other side, take your right hand and thread it under your left arm. Extend your right arm along the floor and let it rest your hand on the floor, palm facing up. Bring your right shoulder down and rest it, along with your right ear, on the floor.

5. Slide the other hand on the floor until it is above your head, palm facing down. Again, if this is too much you can leave your left hand where it is. Take a deep breath in and then exhale. Be sure your neck is relaxed and breathe slowly in and out two more times. Slowly lift your shoulder up and return to starting position.

Take note:

FLOOR ANGELS

Areas stretched: chest, triceps, lats.

1. Lie on the floor facing up with legs straight and arms down by your side. Take a slow, deep breath in and then exhale.

2. Take a breath in while sliding your arms along the floor until they are above your head, palms up, just as if you were making "snow angels" in the snow! Stretch your arms and lengthen your body as much as you are able.

3. Exhale as you bring your arm back down to your sides.

4. Repeat the stretch two or three more times.

Take note:

Once you are comfortable doing this stretch, you can add your legs by sliding your legs apart as you slide your arms up.

CHILD'S POSE

Areas stretched: shoulders, back of neck.

1. Get on the floor on your hands and knees. Your hands should be directly under your shoulders and your knees should be directly under your hips. Take a deep breath in.

2. Lean back as you exhale and bring your glutes down and back to your feet. Lower your torso towards the floor and extend your arms along the floor up over your head. You should be facing the floor and your forehead may be able to come down to the ground. Stretch your arms as much as you can while breathing in deep. Slowly exhale. Take two or three more breaths in this position before returning to the starting position.

Take note:

If your glutes cannot touch your heels, you can place a pillow or rolled up towel between your hamstrings and calves for support.

Be sure to not scrunch up your shoulders when doing this stretch. Neck should be long and shoulders away from the ears.

Lower Body Stretches

BANANA STRETCH

Areas stretched: sides of body including obliques, lats, hips.

1. Lie on the floor, face up towards the ceiling. Stretch your arms up overhead with your hands resting on the floor above you. Stretch your legs out straight. Take a deep, slow breath in.

2. As you exhale, slide your arms and legs along the floor to the left. If you can't do both at the same time, you can slide your arms first and then your legs. You should be in a banana shape and feel a stretch along the right side of your body.

3. Hold this banana shape and breath in and out slowly two or three more times. Return to the starting position.

4. To stretch your other side, slide your arms and legs along the floor to the right. Now you should feel the stretch on your left side. Hold the shape and breath in and out slowly two or three times. Return to the starting position.

Take note:

You can deepen this stretch if you desire. As your arms and legs are sliding to the left, let your left hand grab your right wrist and gently pull. This increases the stretch in your lats and rib cage. If you are sliding to the right, your right hand will grab your left wrist.

To deepen the stretch in your hips and IT band: as your legs slide to the left, cross your right ankle over your left ankle. If your legs are sliding to the right, cross your left ankle over your right one.

WINDSHIELD WIPERS STRETCH

Areas stretched: internal and external hip muscles, tops of quads.

1. Lie on the floor on your back, facing up. Bend your knees so they are pointing up to the ceiling and your feet are flat on the floor, hip width distance apart. Bring your arms out into a T-position.

2. Take a deep breath in. Slowly let both knees fall to the left as you exhale. Inhale as you bring your knees back up. Slowly let both knees now fall to the right and exhale.

3. Repeat the windshield wiper motion, left and right, slowly two or three more times.

Take note:

Only let your legs fall to the side as far as it is comfortable for your hips. Keep your arms out in a T-position to help stabilize your torso as your legs go back and forth.

A variation of this stretch can be done seated. Lean back and support your body with your hands behind you as your legs fall back and forth.

RECLINED FIGURE FOUR

Areas stretched: glutes, hamstrings, hips, lower back.

1. Lie on the floor, facing up. Bend your knees so they are pointing up to the ceiling and your feet are flat on the floor.

2. Bring your right leg up and cross your leg to form a figure four. Your right ankle should be resting on your left leg near your knee. Take a deep breath in and then exhale.

3. Let your hands grab behind your left thigh and bring your left leg towards your chest slowly and gently. Keep both feet flexed to protect your knees. Take a deep inhale and then exhale as you bring your feet back to the ground and uncross your legs.

4. To stretch the other side, bring your left leg up so that your left ankle rests on your right leg. If you can, grab behind your right leg this time and bring it towards you. Inhale slowly and exhale. Uncross your legs and bring both feet back to the ground.

Take note:

Depending on the mobility of your hips, just bringing your ankle up and placing it on top of your other leg may be enough of a stretch for you. Don't feel you have to draw the other leg towards you if you aren't able to.

LYING SPINAL TWIST

Areas stretched: glutes, obliques, chest.

1. Lie on your back on the floor, facing up. Bend your knees so that they are pointing up towards the ceiling and keep your feet next to each other. Bring your arms out into a T-position.

2. Taking a deep breath in. As you exhale, allow both knees to fall to the right until they reach the ground. Your hips should be stacked one on top of the other. If you can, turn your head and look to the left to get a neck stretch.

3. Inhale and then exhale as you bring your knees back up.

4. To stretch the other side, breath in and exhale as both knees now fall to the left until they touch the floor. Again, hips are stacked on top of each other. Look to the right if you can. Take a deep breath and exhale before returning to the starting position.

Take note:

Don't force your knees to the floor. If you cannot twist that far, place a pillow or cushion to the side and let your knees rest on that.

Both shoulders should remain flat on the floor and your chest should be facing the ceiling the whole time. If your shoulder is lifting up, you are twisting too far.

RECLINED BUTTERFLY

Areas stretched: hips, inner thighs, groin muscles.

1. Lie on your back on the floor with your legs straight and your hands by your sides.

2. Take a deep breath in and slowly exhale as you bend the knees and bring the soles of your feet together. Your legs and feet should roughly form a diamond shape. Your knees may or may not touch the floor, depending on the mobility of your hips. Hold this position and breathe in and out slowly two or three times. Return to the starting position.

Take note:

Depending on your flexibility, your feet may be close or far from your groin. Bring your feet to wherever is the most comfortable for you and your inner thigh muscles.

For added stretch, you can slide your arms along the floor up above your head.

Pre-Activity Stretches

Warming up before doing an activity gets your body and muscles ready for action. Just like you warm up a car in cold weather by starting it and letting it heat up to get the fluids moving, it's important to warm up your body to raise your body temperature and get the blood flowing to your muscles. You may be inclined to skip any kind of warm-up in order to get straight to your workout or activity, but you will be missing out on a crucial step and possibly jeopardizing yourself for injury. What are the benefits of warming up and stretching prior to a cardio workout, weight lifting, or sports activity? According to Cronkleton (2019), the benefits include:

- Lessened risk of injury because muscles are relaxed.

- Increased flexibility and ease of movement. Increased range of motion also reduces stress on joints and the tendons that support them.

- Decreased muscle stiffness because muscles are warmed up.

- Greater flow of oxygen and blood throughout your body and muscles because your body temperature has risen while warming up and stretching.

Most of us know to warm up before exercising at home or at the gym, but what about other activities? It's important for the muscles to be warmed up prior to every day activities such as biking, bowling, dancing, gardening, team sports, and even sex. Warming up by gradually increasing your heart rate and breathing allows your body to acclimate to the activity that it will soon be doing.

What is the best way to warm up and stretch prior to our activity? The American Heart Association (2014) recommends the following:

- Walk for five to ten minutes to get the muscles warmed up. An alternative would be to ride a stationary bike or swim for the same amount of time.

- Gradually proceed into your workout by doing whatever you plan on doing for exercise, but at a slower pace. If you are going to run, start off by jogging slowly.

- Incorporate movement into your stretches, but do not bounce. Stretch your entire body, both upper and lower areas.

Don't feel you have to do all the stretches listed in this chapter before your intended activity. Pick a few upper body and a few lower body stretches and do those. Next time, change it up and pick different ones to do.

Upper Body Stretches

CROSS BODY SHOULDER STRETCH

Areas stretched: shoulders, upper back

1. Stand up tall with feet about hips width apart.

2. Bring your left arm up and across your chest to the right side. Support your arm by bending your right arm and letting your left forearm rest in the inside crook of your elbow. Take a deep breath in and then exhale. Return arms to your sides.

3. Next, bring your right arm up and across your chest to the left side. Let your right forearm rest in the inside crook of your other elbow. Breathe in and out. Return arms to your side.

4. Repeat stretches for both arms two or three more times.

Take note:

Alternate support for the arm that is being stretched: stand facing a wall and allow your arm that is crossing your chest to rest between your chest and the wall.

You can also do this stretch while sitting.

OVERHEAD TRICEP STRETCH

Areas stretched: triceps.

1. Stand up tall with your feet about hips width apart. Shrug your shoulders up and then down.

2. Raise your left hand and arm above your head. Bend your left arm and place your left hand on the back of your neck or spine. Use your right hand to gently push your left elbow back as you slide your hand further down, if possible. Take a deep breath in and then exhale. Hold the position for two more breaths in and out. Return the left arm back down to your side.

3. Stretch the other arm by bringing your right hand and arm above your head. Bend the right arm and bring your hand to the back of your neck or spine. Use the other hand to push the right elbow back as your hand reaches further down. Take a deep breath in and then exhale. Hold the position for two more breaths in and out. Return the right arm back down to your side.

4. Repeat the stretch on each arm if desired.

Take note:

Be sure to keep your hips tucked under you so you don't sway and arch out in your lower back. This stretch can also be done while seated.

EAR TO SHOULDER NECK STRETCH

Areas stretched: sides of neck, tops of shoulders.

1. From a standing or sitting position, look straight ahead and relax the shoulders. Shrug the shoulders up and then down.

2. While looking straight ahead, gently tilt the head so the left ear moves towards the top of the left shoulder. Take a deep breath in and then exhale.

3. Gently turn your head so you are now looking at your left armpit. Take a deep breath in and then exhale. Slowly return the head upright.

4. To stretch the other side, look straight ahead and gently tilt the head to the right. Your right ear will move towards the top of your right shoulder. Deep breath in and out.

5. Gently turn your head so your gaze now is towards your right armpit. Take a deep breath in and then exhale. Slowly return the head upright.

Take note:

It's important to be very gentle and careful with your neck, especially if you have any neck problems or pain. Do this stretch slowly and deliberately, pausing when you need to. If looking down towards your armpit is too much for your neck, skip that part.

STANDING CHEST STRETCH

Areas stretched: chest muscles, front of shoulders.

1. Stand up tall with feet hips width apart and arms at your sides.

2. Bring your hands behind you and clasp them together and rest them on your lower back. As you take a breath in, push your chest out as you raise your clasped hands off your lower back and further out behind you. Slowly exhale. Hold the position for two more deep breaths in and out.

3. Return hands to starting position. Repeat the stretch two or three more times if desired.

Take note:

Be sure you do not scrunch up your shoulders as you do this stretch. They should be down and away from your ears and your neck should be kept long and relaxed.

STANDING TORSO TWIST

Areas stretched: abdominals, obliques, spine.

1. With feet about hips width apart, stand up tall with arms at your sides. Lift your arms up and out from your sides to form a T-shape. Take a deep breath in.

2. As you exhale, gently and slowly twist your upper body, including head and arms, to the left. You should be looking to the left and your lower body and hips are still straight ahead. Hold the position and breathe in and out. Return to the starting position.

3. To stretch the other side, breath in as you lift your arms up and out to a T-shape. Exhaling, gently twist your upper body, head, and arms to the right. Again, your hips should still be facing forward and your head should be looking right. Breathe in and out as you hold the position. Return to the starting position.

4. Repeat stretches on both sides two or three more times.

Take note:

Don't be aggressive or jerky as you twist to the left or right. Protect your back and spine by moving slowly and gently.

An alternate arm position is to bend your arms and bring your fingertips to the top of your shoulders as you twist.

Lower Body Stretches

HURDLER HAMSTRING STRETCH

Areas stretched: hamstrings, glutes, hips.

1. Sit on the floor with both legs out straight in front of you. Bend your left leg and bring your foot to the inside of your calf, knee, or thigh.

2. Raise both arms up overhead and take a deep breath in. As you exhale, bend forward at the hip and bring your arms and torso down towards your knee. Depending on your flexibility, you may or may not be able to touch the floor in front of you. Take a deep breath in and exhale. Hold this position for two more breaths in and out. Raise torso and come back up to the starting position.

3. Switch legs by now bending your right leg and bringing your right foot to the inside of your calf, knee, or thigh.

4. Raise both arms up and breathe in. Bend forward towards your knee as you exhale and reach for the floor. Hold this position for two more breaths in and out. Return to the starting position. Repeat the stretch on each side two more times.

Take note:

Remember, don't bounce while doing this stretch and don't force your torso down. Only bend as far as is comfortable for your hamstrings.

STANDING CALF STRETCH

Areas stretched: calves.

1. Standing up tall with feet about 12 to 24 inches away from a wall or sturdy chair, place both hands on the wall or chair.

2. Lift left foot and step it back into a mini lunge while slightly bending the right leg. Press hands against the wall while you bring your left heel down to the floor, if possible. Take a deep breath in and slowly exhale. Bend your left leg to lift the heel off the floor and then try pushing the heel down to the floor again. Return to the starting position.

3. To stretch the other leg, lift the right foot and step back into a mini lunge while slightly bending the other leg. Press your hands against the wall as you bring your right heel down to the floor. Breath in and out. Bend your right leg and lift the heel off the floor and then push the heel down again. Return to the starting position.

4. Repeat the stretch on both sides two more times.

Take note:

Your heel might not touch the floor, and that is okay. The goal here is to stretch your calf muscles to a comfortable point.

QUAD STRETCH

Areas stretched: quads, front of hips.

1. Stand up tall with both feet on the ground. If you need help balancing, you can place one hand on the wall or on the back of a sturdy chair.

2. Bend your left leg behind you and grab your left ankle with your left hand. Bring your heel as close to your glutes as you can without forcing or straining. Take a deep breath in and then exhale. Bring the leg back down to starting position.

3. To stretch the other leg, bend your right leg behind you. Grab your right ankle with your right hand and bring your heel as close as you can to your glutes. Breathe in and out. Bring the leg back down to starting position.

4. Repeat stretches on both legs two more times.

Take note:

Be sure that you don't allow your lower back to arch. Keep the hips tucked under and pelvis facing forward.

If you cannot do this stretch while standing, you can do it while lying on the floor. Laying on your left side, use your right hand to grab your right ankle. Lay on your other side to do the other leg.

SEATED BUTTERFLY

Areas stretched: inner thighs, groin, hips, knees.

1. Sit up tall on the floor with your legs straight out in front of you. Bend your knees out to either side and bring the soles of both feet together.

2. Slide both feet towards you as far as you can, keeping their soles touching. Depending on your flexibility, your knees may be either high off the ground or nearly touching the floor. Your legs make the shape of butterfly wings.

3. Take a deep breath in. While you exhale, bend forward and bring your hands to the ground in front of you as you lean forward slowly. Again, depending on the openness of your hips, you may or may not be able to touch the ground with your hands or lean very far forward. Breathe in and out two more times in this position.

4. Return to the starting position. Do this stretch two more times.

Take note:

If you are able, you can deepen the stretch by allowing your elbows to gently press down on your thighs as you are leaning forward.

Don't round your back as you lean forward. Keep your spine straight, your neck long, and your gaze downwards.

STANDING LUNGE

Areas stretched: hip flexors, quads, calves.

1. Stand up tall with your feet hips width apart. For stability and balance, you can stand next to a wall or sturdy chair for support.

2. Step back with your left foot behind you and bend your right knee. Your right knee should be directly over your right food and bent at a 90 degree angle. Keep your torso upright and do not lean forward. You should feel the stretch in the front of your left hip. Take a deep breath in and then exhale. Hold the position for two more breaths. Return feet to starting position.

3. To stretch the other leg, step back with your right foot while bending your other knee. Now you should feel the stretch in the front of your right hip. Breathe deep in and then out. Hold the position for two more breaths. Return feet to starting position.

4. Repeat the stretch two more times on each side.

Take note:

Do not lean forward during this stretch. Keep your body upright and your pelvis pushed forward to ensure that your hip flexor is engaged and being stretched.
Remember to keep your knee behind your toes so it stays at a 90 degree angle. Letting the knee come forward past your toes puts unnecessary stress on your knee.

Post-Activity Stretches

Stretching and cooling down after participating in an activity is an important way to bring your body back to a normal state. Stopping suddenly after exercising or strenuous activity can cause your blood pressure and heart rate to plummet and make you feel as if you are going to pass out. When we exercise or participate in an activity that gets our heart rate up, our blood is pumping and our blood vessels are dilated to deliver blood and oxygen to our muscles. Coming to a sudden stop can cause a feeling of sickness and lightheadedness. Gradually ceasing the activity helps the body shift to a decrease in movement and exertion.

It is beneficial to stretch as the body is cooling down after exercise or prolonged activity. Your muscles are still warm and so are your joints and tendons. Stretching while still warm allows the muscles to stretch further and deeper, leading to increased flexibility and mobility. It is also good to stretch after activity to prevent the buildup of lactic acid in the muscles. Lactic acid builds up in muscles when there is not enough oxygen getting to the muscles. The result is stiffness and soreness in the muscles that can last for days. Stretching, as well as drinking plenty of water, helps prevent lactic acid build up (Cronkleton, 2018) by encouraging circulation and relieving muscle tension.

What is the best way to cool down and stretch, post-activity? According to the American Heart Association (2014), you should:

- Walk until your heart rate comes down (ideally below 120 beats per minute), about five minutes.

- Stretch the entire body, both upper and lower, and hold stretches for several breaths, about 30 seconds.

- Stretch deeply but not to the point of pain. Never bounce while stretching.

Cooling down and stretching after exercise and activity allows our bodies to recover and our heart rate and blood pressure to gradually return to what they were before we started our activity. Stretching while muscles are warm also prevents the blood from pooling in our lower body or other extremities after exercising. Plus, stretching after exercise or any activity feels good!

Upper Body Stretches

WRIST ROTATION BICEP STRETCH

Areas stretched: biceps, thumb, shoulder.

1. Stand up tall with your feet about hips width apart. Raise your arms out and away from your sides into a T position.

2. With your palms facing forward, make each hand into a fist leaving the thumb free and pointed up. You will be making the "thumbs up" sign with both hands! Take a deep breath in and then exhale.

3. Now, rotate your wrists and arms so that your thumbs are pointing towards the floor. You will now be making the "thumbs down" sign with both hands. Breath in and out.

4. Repeat the stretch two or three more times going from thumbs up to thumbs down slowly and breathing naturally.

Take note:

Don't let your shoulders round and don't let your chest collapse inwards while doing this stretch. Keep your chest out and pushed forward for good posture.

You can do this stretch while seated.

SHOULDER ROLLS

Areas stretched: shoulders including trapezius muscles.

1. Stand up tall with feet about hips width apart and arms hanging down by your sides.

2. Slowly raise your shoulders up towards your ears and then roll them back, squeezing your shoulder blades together. Breathing naturally, roll the shoulders up and back three to five more times. Return shoulders to the starting position.

3. Now roll the shoulders the other way by slowly raising them up towards your ears and roll them forward while rounding your upper back. Breathe naturally and continue to roll the shoulders up and forward three to five more times. Return shoulders to the starting position.

Take note:

This stretch can be done any time your neck and shoulders are starting to feel tense. You can also do this stretch while sitting.

EAGLE ARMS POSE

Areas stretched: shoulders, upper back, triceps.

1. From a standing or sitting position, bring both arms out in front of you and bend them so the elbows form a 90 degree angle.

2. Cross the forearms so that the right elbow is under the left elbow and the backs of your hands are touching each other. Raise your arms so that your elbows are about shoulder height. Take a deep breath in and then exhale. You should feel this stretch all across your upper back and shoulders. Slowly uncross forearms and return arms to your sides.

3. To stretch the other way, bring your arms out in front of you and bend them again. Cross forearms this time so that your left elbow is under your right one. Raise your elbows to about shoulder height and breathe deeply in and out. Slowly uncross forearms and return arms to your sides.

4. Repeat this stretch two or three more times.

Take note:

Depending on the size of your arms and your chest, you may or may not be able to cross your forearms and get one elbow under the other. It is perfectly okay to just bring the forearms together and raise your elbows to shoulder height. Be sure to keep your shoulders down and away from your ears. Don't scrunch up! If you want to deepen the stretch, instead of just the backs of your hands touching each other, do another cross at the wrists and try to get your palms to touch each other.

SUPERMAN STRETCH

Areas stretched: upper back, shoulders, abdominals, spinal muscles, lower back, glutes.

1. Lie on the floor, face and belly down, with arms out in front of you and legs straight.

2. Take a deep breath in and slowly raise your arms and legs off the floor a few inches and draw in your belly button. You should feel a contraction in your lower back and your body should look as if you are flying through the air like a superhero! Exhale and slowly lower your arms and legs to the ground.

3. Repeat the stretch two or three more times.

Take note:

Keep your neck straight and look down at the ground, not straight ahead of you as that will put too much pressure on the neck.

Lift your arms and legs only to where it is comfortable. If lifting both is too hard, just lift your arms.

LYING PECTORAL STRETCH

Areas stretched: pectoral and chest muscles.

1. Lie on the floor face and belly down. Legs should be straight and arms extended straight out to the sides away from your body.

2. Bend your left arm and bring your left hand on the floor just under your left shoulder. Take a deep breath in and while exhaling push into your left hand as you roll onto your right hip. Keep your right arm straight and extended out. You should feel the stretch in the right chest area. Hold this position for two more breaths in and out. Roll back to the starting position.

3. To stretch the other side, bend your right arm and bring your right hand under your right shoulder. Breathe in and exhale as you push into your right hand and roll onto your left hip. Your left arm should be straight and extended. Roll back down to the starting position.

4. Repeat this stretch on both sides two more times.

Take note:

Roll to the side only as far as it is comfortable for you. As you become more accustomed to the stretch, you will be able to roll farther.

Lower Body Stretches

LYING HAMSTRING STRETCH

Areas Stretched: hamstrings, glutes.

1. Lie down on the floor with legs straight and arms down by your sides.

2. Raise your left leg and with both hands grab the back of your calf, knee, or thigh to support it. Take a deep breath in, and then exhale. Hold the position for two more breaths and gently bring your leg closer to your body, only if it is comfortable. Lower the leg back to the floor.

3. Stretch the other leg by bringing your right leg up and with both hands grab your leg where you can. Breath in deeply and then exhale. Hold the position for two more breaths and attempt to gently bring your leg closer to your body. Lower the leg back to the floor.

4. Repeat the stretch on each side two more times.

Take note:

Keep your head and upper back on the floor as you raise your leg to avoid straining your neck. If you are not able to grab your leg with both hands, an alternative is to do this stretch lying next to a wall, bed, or sofa where you can support the lifted leg.

BRIDGE POSE

Areas stretched: glutes, abdominals, hamstrings.

1. Lie down on the floor on your back with your arms by your sides. Bend your knees so they are pointing up to the ceiling and bring the back of your heels as close to your glutes as you can.

2. Take a deep breath in and exhale as you push your feet into the floor and lift your hips up and towards the ceiling. There should be a diagonal line from your shoulders to your knees. Hold the position while breathing normally for 30 seconds. If you can't hold your hips up that long, it is okay. Lower hips back down to the floor gently.

3. Repeat the stretch four or five more times.

Take note:

Don't raise your hips too high. You want to avoid hyperextending your lower back. Your shoulders and hips should be in a line.

Maintain good form when doing this stretch. It's better to hold the position for a shorter amount of time but correctly rather than holding it for 30 seconds incorrectly.

HAPPY BABY

Areas stretches: inner thighs, hamstrings, groin, lower back, hips.

1. Lie on the floor on your back. Bend your knees and bring them towards you so your feet are facing up towards the ceiling.

2. Keep your head on the mat as you reach your hands up to grab your feet. You can grab the outer edge or inside arch of your feet, whichever is more comfortable for you. Let your knees fall away from each other and try to bring your knees to your armpits.

3. Gently rock from side to side, like a happy baby, while keeping your feet flexed. Breathe normally throughout the stretch. You can hold this stretch for several breaths, or whatever is comfortable for you.

Take note:

Keep your head and shoulders on the floor for the entire stretch. Avoid straining your neck. If you cannot grab your feet without lifting your head or shoulders, try grabbing onto your ankles or shins instead.

SQUARE POSE

Areas stretched: hips, inner thighs, spine.

1. Sit on the floor. Bend your left leg on the floor in front of you so that your knee faces towards the left. Bend your right leg and put your right shin on top of your left. You should be sitting cross legged with your right leg directly on top of your left, shins stacked. Breathe in deep and then exhale. Hold this position for two or three more breaths.

2. To stretch the other hip, change the cross of your legs with your left leg on top this time. Left shin should be stacked directly on top of the right one. Hold this position for two or three more breaths.

Take note:

If it is hard for you to sit upright in this position, place a blanket or towel under your tailbone for support.

To deepen this stretch, fold your upper body forward using your hands on the floor for support. You can either keep your spine straight and long or round your back for a more passive pose.

KNEE TO OPPOSITE SHOULDER IT BAND STRETCH

Areas stretched: iliotibial (IT) band.

1. Lie on your back on the floor with your legs straight and arms by your sides.

2. Bend and raise your left knee towards you, grabbing behind your knee with both hands. Gently bring your knee towards the right shoulder. You should feel the stretch on the outside of your left hip and thigh where the IT band runs. Take a deep breath in and out. Hold the position for two or three more breaths. Gently lower the leg back to the starting position.

3. To stretch the other leg, raise and bend your right leg. Grab behind your knee and gently bring your right knee towards your left shoulder. Breathe deeply in and then exhale. Hold the position for two or three more breaths. Gently lower the leg and return to the starting position.

4. Repeat the stretch on both legs two more times.

Take note:

A tight IT band can cause pain at the knee and hip joints, so go slowly and carefully when doing this stretch. Don't jerk on your knee at any time.

Keep your head and shoulders on the floor to avoid any neck strain.

Target Area Stretches

In the previous chapters, we have concentrated on the large muscles of the upper and lower body. These are the muscles that contribute to our daily movement and mobility. There are many other muscles that can be stretched to relieve pain or to increase flexibility in a targeted area of the body. In this chapter, we will learn some stretches that work on some of the smaller, but no less important, areas that can benefit from a stretching routine.

The extremities, namely the hands and feet, are used daily and can become tight or stiff. Stretching the fingers, hands, and wrists helps with fine motor skills and mobility to do simple tasks like holding small items, writing, buttoning clothing, eating, using scissors, and even typing. The small muscles in our hands were designed to accomplish these fine motor skills. As we grow older, we sometimes find that our ability to do some of these skills diminishes because of joint stiffness and a loss of muscle flexibility. By doing a few easy stretches every day, we keep our joints and muscles moving and limber, allowing us to continue doing the activities that call for fine motor control.

Stretching the toes, feet, and ankles keeps us on our feet, literally. If you have ever experienced foot or ankle pain, you know how debilitating that can be to physical movement and even mental health. Our feet are subjected to daily pressure which is sometimes made worse by inflammation, conditions like plantar fasciitis, and even ill-fitting shoes. The benefits of stretching the big muscles in our arms and legs apply also to the small muscles in our feet. Increased blood flow and circulation brings oxygen to the muscles in our feet and allows us to stretch the muscles and elongate them, reducing pain and stiffness. The increased flexibility in our feet also aids us in our balance. This helps prevent falls due to imbalance.

These targeted areas are also areas that are prone to arthritis and other joint conditions, so if you have challenges with that check with your doctor, chiropractor, or health provider before doing these stretches. As always, use common sense and discontinue any stretch that causes pain at any time.

Upper Body Stretches

HAND AND FINGER TENDON GLIDE

Areas stretched: tendons in the hands and fingers

1. With both hands in front of you and palms facing each other, straighten the fingers and thumbs. Slowly bend just the fingers until the fingertips touch the upper part of your palms. Hold the position for 30 seconds. Straighten fingers slowly.

2. Next, bend fingers until the fingertips touch the middle of the palms. Make a fist by bringing thumbs over the fingers. Hold the position for 30 seconds. Slowly straighten fingers and thumbs.

3. Finally, keep fingers straight and bend at the knuckle to bring fingertips down towards the bottom or meaty part of the palms. Hold the position for 30 seconds. Bring fingers back to starting position.

4. Repeat the three stretches a few more times. Breathe normally throughout the stretching.

Take note:

Depending on your finger and hand mobility, these exercises may be difficult for one or both hands. You can also do these stretches one hand at a time.

Don't hold your breath or clench your jaw while doing these stretches. It can sometimes happen when we are focused and intent, so just be aware!

WRIST FLEXOR AND EXTENSOR STRETCH

Areas stretched: wrists, forearms.

1. From a seated position, rest your left forearm on a table or countertop so that your elbow forms a 90 degree angle. Position yourself so that your left arm is next to your body with your left hand facing down and wrist hanging over the edge of the table. Slowly lower your hand so that your palm is now facing you and your fingertips are pointing towards the floor.

2. Slowly raise your hand so that your palm is now facing away from you and your fingertips are pointing towards the ceiling. Do this stretch both ways two more times, breathing normally while stretching.

3. Change positions so that now your right forearm is resting on the table with your right hand facing down and wrist over the edge. Lower your right hand slowly so your palm is facing you and your fingertips are pointing towards the floor.

4. Raise your hand slowly until your right palm is facing away from you and fingertips are pointing at the ceiling. Stretch both ways two more times while breathing normally.

Take note:

If needed, you can place a folded or rolled hand towel under your forearm for extra padding and support.

A variation of this stretch is to form your hand into a fist with your thumb over your fingers. Lower and raise your fist slowly.

WRIST ULNAR AND RADIAL STRETCH

Areas stretched: wrists, forearms.

1. From a seated position, rest your left forearm on a table so that your elbow forms a 90 degree angle. Bring your left arm next to your body with your thumb and fingertips straight ahead with your palm facing inward. Slowly lower your wrist and hand toward the floor and then bring it up straight ahead and slightly towards the ceiling if possible, going through the full range of motion. Breathe normally as you repeat this stretch two more times.

2. To stretch the other side, change positions so that your right forearm is resting on the table. With your right arm next to your body and fingertips straight ahead, face your palm inward. Slowly move your hand and wrist up toward the ceiling and down toward the floor, through the full range of motion. Repeat the stretch two more times.

Take note:

This stretch uses different muscles in the wrist and forearm and you may not have the same range of flexibility as you do with other wrist stretches.

BUTTERFLY WINGS UPPER BACK STRETCH

Areas stretched: upper back including rhomboids, upper chest including pecs.

1. From

2. a standing or seated position, lift both arms and bend at the elbows. Allow the fingertips to touch the shoulders, left hand touches left shoulder and right hand touches right shoulder. These form the "butterfly wings."

3. Take a deep breath in. As you exhale, bring your elbows together out in front of you and try to touch them together. Be sure to keep your fingertips on your shoulders.

4. Gently bring elbows back out to sides and slightly behind you, if possible. Repeat the stretch both ways two or three more times, exhaling as you bring your elbows together.

Take note:

Depending on the size of your chest and your flexibility, you may or may not be able to touch your elbows together. It's okay if they don't touch. Your upper back will still experience a stretch.

Areas stretched: abdominals.

1. Lie on the floor, face down, with your feet pointing away from you. Place your hands directly under your shoulders.

2. Take a deep breath in. As you exhale, press down through your hands to raise your upper torso off the floor. Keep shoulders down and away from your ears while keeping your neck long. Hips and legs should remain on the floor. Breathe in and out once more and slowly lower your torso back down to the floor.

3. Repeat this stretch two or three more times, going slowly.

Take note:

Do not do this stretch if you have any back issues or severe back pain.

Only lift up your torso as far as it is comfortable for you.

Lower Body Stretches

TOE RAISES, POINTS, AND CURLS

Areas stretched: toes, feet, ankles.

1. From a seated position in a chair, place both feet flat on the floor. Keeping toes and balls of the feet on the floor, raise both heels so they are off the floor as high as you can get them. Hold the position for 15 to 30 seconds.

2. Next, point your toes, ballerina style, so that only the tips of your big toes (and possibly your second toes) are on the ground. Hold the position for 15 to 30 seconds.

3. Finally, curl your toes towards the soles of your feet. Now the tops of your toes should be on the ground and you feel the stretch in the front of your ankles. Hold the position for 15 to 30 seconds. Return feet to the starting position.

4. Repeat the stretches two or three more times.

Take note:

If you have had any foot surgery, check with your doctor before doing these stretches.

Breathe normally while doing these stretches and keep your shoulders down and relaxed. If you feel any pain while doing the stretches, immediately stop.

TOE EXTENSION OR FOOT FLEX

Areas stretched: heels, ankles.

1. From a seated position, bring your left ankle up and place it on top of your right knee. Grab your left toes with your left hand and gently pull them up towards your ankle. You should feel the stretch in your heel and back of the ankle. Hold for two breaths in and out and return foot to the starting position.

2. To stretch the other foot, bring your right ankle up and place it on top of your left knee. Use your right hand to grab your right toes and gently pull them towards your ankle. Hold the position for two breaths and return foot to the starting position.

3. Repeat stretches on both feet two or three more times.

Take note:

This stretch is helpful if you have plantar fasciitis or heel pain.

If you cannot bring your ankle up to your knee, you can do this stretch by crossing your legs and stretching the foot by bringing your toes up towards your calf.

ANKLE ALPHABET

Areas stretched: ankles, calves.

1. Sit up straight on the floor with legs straight out in front of you. Your hands can be on the floor for support and balance.

2. Place a pillow or rolled up towel under your left calf so that your left foot and ankle are off the floor. Point your left foot and draw the letter A with your toes. Then draw the letter B, the letter C, and so forth. After you have completed the alphabet, switch the pillow to the other calf.

3. With your right calf supported by the pillow and right foot and ankle off the floor, point your right foot and draw the alphabet with your toes.

Take note:

Don't worry if you find it hard to get through the entire alphabet the first few times. As you do this stretch regularly, your ankles will get stronger and your range of motion will increase.

This stretch can also be done sitting in a chair.

KNEELING SHIN STRETCH

Areas stretched: shins.

1. Kneel on the floor or a padded mat, with your legs bent and feet behind you. Your knees should be touching each other. Slowly lower your buttocks and sit them down on the soles of your feet. Hold this position for two or three breaths in and out. Slowly come back up to the starting position.

2. Repeat the stretch two or three more times.

Take note:

Be sure your buttocks do not fall between your feet when you lower down. Keep your knees and feet together.

If your knees do not allow you to sit all the way back onto your feet, come part way

down or as far as you can. You may need to support yourself with hands on the floor or holding onto a sturdy chair.

HIP ROTATIONS

Areas stretched: hips.

1. Stand up tall with feet a little wider than hips width apart. Place your hands on your hips.

2. Keeping your feet firmly on the ground, move your hips clockwise in a large circle from one side, to the front, to the other side, and to the back. Make five large circles going in the same direction. Return to the starting position.

3. Now move your hips counterclockwise, going in the other direction, in a large circle. Make five large circles and then return to the starting position.

4. Repeat the hip rotations, going both ways, two or three more times.

Take note:

Breathe normally while doing this stretch. Be sure that you are making large enough circles so that your hips are being stretched.

Don't lock your knees but keep them slightly bent.

Conclusion

Stretching is an important part of maintaining our body and general well-being as we progress into our later years of life. As we have learned throughout this book, stretching is for everyone, not just competitive athletes and professional dancers. A regular stretching routine can be done anywhere and at any time of the day. Stretching before and after exercise and strenuous activity is a no-brainer, but we saw that stretching in the morning and in the evening are not only beneficial but help us shift into and out of the events of our day.

There are many wrong ways to stretch that can actually hurt instead of help our bodies, so we learned some things to avoid. Remembering to first warm up before stretching is crucial as well as being careful to not bounce while stretching. Incorporating a variety of stretches is important to keep our muscles from any imbalances that may occur because of doing the same stretches again and again. The goal is muscle strength as well as symmetry. While we do want to stretch to the point of muscle tension, we have to stop before any stretch becomes painful because this is detrimental to our goal of flexibility and increased range of motion.

One of the goals in putting together this book of stretches was to provide a resource for older adults. Having a book that you can turn to again and again as you embark on a journey to better health through stretching is helpful. It is also convenient to have these stretches in one volume. The stretches in each chapter can be mixed and matched to fit your personal fitness goal and individual needs. As was mentioned previously, stretching is not a quick fix, but rather a lifestyle choice. Of the factors that contribute to our biological age, or the age at which our body functions, physical activity is one of the factors that we can easily control and easily pursue. While our chronological age, or how many years we have lived on this planet, can never change, our biological age can. The mobility and flexibility of our bodies help our biological age to always be younger than our natural born years.

All the best to you and to your health! If you enjoyed this book, please feel free to recommend it and leave a review on Amazon.

Scan The QR Code to Leave a Review:

I trust you will experience excellent health and well-being on the long road of life that lies before you and wish you my very best. Thank you for letting me share my knowledge with you.

-Baz Thompson

Balance Exercises for Seniors

Simple Movements to Improve Posture, Decrease Back Pain, and Prevent Injury After 60

Baz Thompson

Introduction

Aging is not lost youth but a new stage of opportunity and strength.
—Betty Freidan

Welcome to the initial step in regaining and maintaining your balance! You may be currently having stability issues, recovering from an injury, or just taking preventative steps to keep physically strong and well balanced. We will walk on this journey together to learn about our bodies, discover how to stay strong and stable as our bodies age, and employ simple steps to keep, or recover, our balance.

The Vestibular Disorders Association defines balance this way:

Balance is the ability to maintain the body's center of mass over its base of support. A properly functioning balance system allows humans to see clearly while moving, identify orientation with respect to gravity, determine direction and speed of movement, and make automatic postural adjustments to maintain posture and stability in various conditions and activities. (Watson, et al., n.d.).

In other words, balance is the capability to remain stable and upright. When we think of balance, certain things come to mind, such as: a person learning to ride a unicycle, a young gymnast walking on a balance beam, or a trapeze artist walking on a tightrope. These activities all involve a good deal of balance and may be things some people are not ever able to do. But balance is more than circus tricks and gymnastic feats. It is an important and vital part of functioning in our everyday lives. Some ways that we use balance in our daily life include:

- Getting up out of bed
- Walking across the room
- Sitting down in a chair
- Going up and down stairs
- Getting in and out of cars
- Carrying bags and packages
- Turning to look behind you
- Stepping aside to let others pass you
- Reaching forward to grasp something

Our body's natural ability to balance starts to slowly diminish once we reach our mid-40's. As we age, things that contribute to the decline in balance include vision problems, inner ear issues, and other injuries or illnesses. One of the overlooked causes of the loss of balance, however, is inactivity. When older adults become sedentary and lose muscular strength in their core, upper body, and lower body, a loss of balance follows. The good news is balance can be regained and maintained with regular exercise and training. All ages can improve their balance and become stronger, but those who are over 40 years old should incorporate balance exercises into their regular activity routine.

BENEFITS OF EXERCISE

Balance exercises ought to be done regularly, along with cardio, weights, and stretching, as part of a fitness and preventative program. Why exercise? We all know that regular exercise is good for you, but it is especially important as we age. The Surgeon General reports that as we age, we become less active. A third of all men and half of all women engage in no physical activity by the time they are 75 years old (CDC, 2019). This reduced activity leads to a loss of stamina and strength.

MISCONCEPTIONS

First, some misconceptions about exercise should be addressed. Perhaps you have heard people say these or have even thought about them yourself. Common misconceptions about exercise include:

- I'm too old. If you are still alive, you aren't too old to start an exercise program. Older adults who have either never exercised or are just getting back into exercising again after years of inactivity quickly show improvement in their physical and mental capacities by participating in regular movement and exertion.

- I'm not the athlete I was. For those who were very active or competitive athletes in their youth, it can be disheartening to not have the ability or strength to do what they once were able to do. By remembering that we all are getting older, we can be realistic about expectations. Our bodies change over time and certain abilities decline with age, but a sense of satisfaction and enjoyment can still be had by participating in age-appropriate activities.

- I will get old anyway. Exercise doesn't stop us from getting older, but it does help us look and feel younger. Regular physical activity boosts energy, helps maintain or lose weight, and bolsters the immune system. By staying healthy, we get to enjoy longer life and stay independent while living it.

- I'm disabled or in ill health. If this is your situation, you have extra challenges in getting movement into your life. However, starting off slowly and gently with what you are able to do, such as stretching or other gentle activities like chair yoga, can get you on a path that eventually will allow you to do more as you get stronger. Getting in some type of consistent and gentle physical activity will also help you manage aches and pains better.

ADVANTAGES OF EXERCISE

There are advantages to starting and keeping consistent with an exercise plan. The specific benefits that come from exercising include:

- Prevention of disease. Exercise boosts the immune system of the body and helps ward off illnesses such as colds and flus, but it also can help prevent more serious conditions such as heart disease, high blood pressure, and diabetes. Physical activity such as walking, swimming, and biking are all good ways to get moving. Activities such as bowling, dancing, tennis, and golf are some non-impact sports that are suitable for aging adults.

- Promotion of good mental health. Exercise and prolonged activities cause the body to produce the feel-good hormones called endorphins. When released into our body systems, these hormones relieve stress and promote a sense of happiness and well-being. Getting in some physical activity also results in better and deeper sleep at night. Many older adults have trouble sleeping, sometimes because of inactivity.

- Improvement of cognitive function. Because physical activity requires the use of large, small, and fine motor skills, it stimulates cognitive functioning in the brain. The risk of dementia and other age-related decline in cognitive abilities increases as we age but the likelihood of it happening can be reduced with regular exercise.

- Lessened fall risks. Older adults take longer to recover from injuries resulting from a fall, and that can lead to a loss of independence. Exercise increases the body's strength, agility, and flexibility, all of which are needed to help prevent falls.

- Engagement with others. Maintaining ties to groups of friends or the local community is important as we age to help prevent isolation as well as feelings of depression and loneliness. By exercising at a gym or with others, we can make physical exercise a fun and social activity.

TYPES OF EXERCISE

Finding a form of physical activity that you enjoy is a key component to maintaining consistency in the long-term. Exercise does not need to be strenuous to be effective. Spending hours at the gym on the treadmill or lifting heavy weights is not realistic or helpful once we hit the senior years. But some type of physical exertion is important and should be done daily or at least five days a week, according to the U.S. Department of Health and Human Services (Elsawy and Higgens, 2010).

The areas of exercise that ought to be included are:

- Cardiovascular. Sometimes simply called cardio, this type of exercise uses the large muscle groups in your body and elevates the heart rate. Practiced regularly, it lessens fatigue and decreases shortness of breath along with strengthening the heart.

- Examples include: cycling, dancing, hiking, rowing, stair climbing, swimming, tennis, and walking.

- ○ Recommended time: 150 minutes of moderate-intensity aerobic activity (30 minutes, five days a week) or 75 minutes of vigorous-intensity aerobic activity (20 minutes, five days a week).

- ○ Strength Training. This type of exercise involves lifting or pushing against something with resistance. The repetitive motion and resistance helps to build bone mass, muscle, and strength.

- ○ Examples include: hand held or free weights, weight machines, resistance bands, or your own body weight.

- ○ Recommended time: strength training of all the major muscle groups two days a week.

- ○ Flexibility. Keeping your muscles and joints limber and able to move freely through a full range of motion is the goal of flexibility exercises. It has been said that *"motion is lotion"* when it comes to joint health.

- ○ Examples include: calisthenics, yoga, tai chi, and stretching.

- ○ Recommended time: 10 minutes, two days a week.

- ○ Balance Exercises. Starting in our mid-40's, our balance abilities start to slowly decline. However, practicing and training our balance with regular exercises can help regain and maintain our equilibrium and stability.

- ○ Examples include: seated exercises, standing exercises, walking, core exercises, and vestibular exercises that all target balance and strength.

- ○ Recommended time: 10 minutes, five days a week.

EXERCISES IN THIS BOOK

For the remainder of this book, we will be concentrating on the last type of exercise; balance exercises. The goal is to inform you, the reader, on the whys and hows of balance exercises as well as give you 50 exercises that you can start doing today to work on your equilibrium and stability. It is never too early, or too late, to start building your ability to balance.

- ○ In Chapter 1, we will take a look at how our brain keeps our body in balance as well as some statistics on losing your balance and what the results of that are long-term. We will also talk about the risk factors for falls and how to reduce them. At the end of the chapter, there is a list of balance tests for you to perform to gauge how you are doing in terms of balance.

- ○ Chapter 2 concentrates on seated balance exercises. These exercises only require a sturdy chair and will work on building stability from a seated position.

- ○ Standing balance exercises are outlined in Chapter 3. Working on strength and steadiness while in a standing position is what we focus on in this chapter.

- ○ In Chapter 4, we will take a look at adding movement in with some standing balance exercises. These walking exercises require some multitasking and will help build confidence in your ability to balance while walking.

- ○ Chapter 5 targets core strength. Our abdominal and back muscles are key to our overall capacity for good balance, so we will spotlight the ways we can build power in our core.

- ○ The vestibular system is addressed in Chapter 6. We focus here on exercises that retrain our brain, eyes, and inner ear for good equilibrium.

- ○ In Chapter 7, we include some tailored workout routines that incorporate the exercises found in the previous chapters. It is a good starting point for a month's worth of weekly routines that include core strength, leg strength, vestibular strength, and walking.

HOW TO USE THIS BOOK

Not only will you learn important information about your body and the subject of balance, you will also find 50 practical exercises that you can start using right away. Look at this book as a balance guidebook that you can refer back to again and again.

In each of the chapters containing exercises, the individual moves will include the amount of time each exercise takes to complete, the areas of the body that you are working on, and detailed directions on how to do the exercise. Many exercises will include instructions on how to take the move to the next level and make it more challenging once you have gotten stronger and more stable. At the end of each exercise will be reminders on what to take note of and cautions to remember. Illustrations that accompany each exercise will show each move done correctly, and will guide you and help you to position your head, body, arms, legs, and feet accordingly. As mentioned previously, you can work through each exercise in this book, one at a time, or follow the exercise plans that are included towards the end of the book. Find a way for these exercises to work for you, then stick with it. You can achieve better balance and equilibrium with some effort!

If you are starting any new type of activity, you are encouraged to consult with your doctor prior to embarking on any exercise program.

Getting older is inevitable for us all, but losing our balance and experiencing falls do not have to go along with aging. By becoming educated on our bodies, learning to make the changes we need to, deciding to take steps to better health, and then finally following through with our decisions with action, we can all enjoy the second half of our lives with good health and vitality.

My hope and goal is that you will find this book a helpful tool as you work on regaining and maintaining good balance to prevent falls and enhance your overall well being. **Are you ready? Let's get your fitness education and training started!**

The Importance of Balance

Getting old is like climbing a mountain; you get a little out of breath, but the view is much better!

—Ingmar Bergman

It has been said that aging is not for the faint of heart. If we consider the importance of balance, we could add that aging is also not for those who lose their balance. Remaining strong and stable is crucial to living a vibrant and active life as you approach your 60s, 70s, 80s, and beyond. Balance and stability in our bodies helps us to maintain our physical health and do the things we enjoy.

What happens, however, when we have a loss in the ability to keep our good balance? In this chapter, we will learn about the three body systems that contribute to our balance. We will also look at the biggest consequence when we no longer have good balance, what increases our risks for falling, and what can be done to prevent it. We will also learn how to test our balance at home.

THE SCIENCE OF BALANCE

Mike was a car enthusiast who enjoyed taking his vintage convertible out for a drive every Sunday. Sometimes, he would take along one of his grandkids and they would stop for ice cream. The convertible was parked in his extra car garage. To get there, Mike would walk from his concrete driveway, across the grass in his side yard, and onto a gravel path. Although he was in his late sixties, Mike didn't have any problems transitioning from one walking surface to the next because he had good balance and a stable core. His Aston-Martin was sleek, fast, and sat low to the ground, making it a fun car to drive with the top down. Mike easily got in and out of the driver's seat because his legs and core were strong.

It is easy to take good balance for granted. But someone with impaired balance would have had a difficult time in the scenario above. Stumbling over surface transitions and having trouble squatting up and down into a lowered seat can be tiring and even dangerous for a person who struggles with balance issues.

THE HOWS OF BALANCE

How does our body maintain balance and equilibrium? There are three main body systems that contribute to our overall balance. These include sensory input from three areas of our bodies, the processing of that input, and our bodies reaction to the input.

SENSORY INPUT

Our brains receive information from all parts of our bodies. For balance, the brain particularly looks at the nerve impulses received from the eyes, the ears, and the muscles and joints in our arms and legs.

- ○ Visual. The rods and cones in our eyes send messages to the the brain to help it determine where our bodies are in relation to our surroundings. These visual cues help us to approach or avoid things in our path and keep us aligned.

- ○ Touch. Sensors in our skin, muscles, and joints relay information so that our brain knows when we are taking a step forward, which way our head is turned, and where our body is in the space we are occupying.

- ○ Vestibular. The inner canals and working of our ears make up the majority of the vestibular system. It contributes to the awareness of equilibrium and motion. The impulses that the sensors send to the brain allows us to know if we are standing, lying down, or turning, among other things.

INTEGRATION OF INPUT

The coming together of all the input received in the brain is broken down and assigned to certain parts of the brain. The brain stem combines and sorts information from the senses.

- ○ Cerebellum. Called the coordination center of the brain, the cerebellum regulates posture and balance. It relies on automatic reactions and previous history from repeated exposure to certain actions. This is the part of the brain that helps a racquetball player know what kind of balance they will need to serve the ball.

- ○ Cerebral cortex. This thinking and memory command center of the brain contributes to memory and critical thinking, like decision making. Stored information in this area helps a person remember that walking on a rainy street requires extra caution because of slip hazards and slick surfaces.

MOTOR INPUT

Finally, the brain stem again comes into the picture. It sends messages to all areas of the body and tells it what to do to maintain balance. Some reflexes include:

- ○ Eye reflex. Called the vestibulo-ocular reflex, this automatic function of our eyes is triggered by the information coming from the brain. It allows your gaze to remain steady, even if your head is moving from side to side or up and down.

- ○ Motor impulses. These oversee eye movements and make body adjustments. With the information from the brain, your muscles and joints can move in the way they need to based on information from your eyes. If you have ever seen a dancer or ice skater twirl around and around repeatedly while keeping their balance, you have seen this motor impulse in action.

- ○

FEAR OF FALLING

Marilyn was a mother and grandmother who loved to spend time with her kids and grandchildren on a regular basis. She loved to bake with her grandkids and take them to the movies. At one time, Marilyn was an avid tennis player, but because she was now in her early seventies, she didn't play as much tennis as she used to. She also didn't feel like going to the gym anymore because the exercise classes were just too hard for her. Her joints became more creaky and her arthritis flared up from time to time, but overall she was doing okay. She was in the kitchen one day, reaching for a baking pan that was at the back of the shelf, when she lost her balance and fell. As she was falling, she hit her head on the edge of the countertop before landing on her hip on the kitchen tile flooring. She wound up with stitches for the cut on her forehead and a broken hip that required surgery. Because of the injuries she sustained, Marilyn not only lost her mobility, but lost some of her independence to drive and get around on her own as well.

Falls are not a normal part of aging. Yet, every year, millions of older adults lose their balance, fall, and injure themselves. The Center for Disease Control (CDC) statistics related to falls are sobering. They include:

- One-fourth of adults over 65 years old fall each year.
- Once you fall, your chance for falling again doubles.
- Emergency rooms across the nation see over three million older adults for injuries related to falls and 800,000 of those are hospitalized because of head or hip injuries that are a result from their fall.
- One-fifth of falls cause serious injury like head trauma or broken bones.
- Traumatic brain injuries are most commonly caused by a fall.
- Over 95 percent of hip fractures are the result of a fall (CDC, 2019).

While falls may not always cause serious injury, twenty percent of the time, the injuries are bad enough that it becomes difficult for the injured person to accomplish everyday activities, drive, or live independently.

FALL RISK FACTORS

While anyone can accidentally trip and fall, there are certain conditions that make it more likely for you to fall. These risk factors include:

- Vision problems. Because of age and either injury or illness, we can experience problems with our vision. Not being able to see objects at our feet or in our pathway can cause us to stumble over them and potentially fall.
- Foot pain. Having foot pain can occur from either injury to the foot or simply from ill-fitting shoes that lack support and grip. To maintain balance, we need the sensory feedback from our feet, ankles, knees, and hips.
- Prescription and over-the-counter medications. Doctor prescribed medications can sometimes cause dizziness or drowsiness, especially pain medication, seda-

tives, tranquilizers, and antidepressants. OTC medications such as antihistamines, cough syrups, and cold medicines can also affect your steadiness on your feet.

○ Vitamin D deficiency. The relationship between vitamin D and good bone health is well established. There is also some evidence that when vitamin D levels fall below a certain point in the body, muscle functioning is decreased and the risk for falls increases (Akdeniz et al., 2016).

○ Trip hazards in the home. Uneven steps, loose carpeting or floor tiles, electrical cords, and throw rugs are all common trip hazards at home. Poor or dim lighting, items left on the floor, and water or other liquid that has spilled on the floor are other dangers that can contribute to falls.

○ Core and lower body weakness. Older adults can sometimes become fearful of falling and cut back on their physical activities. Unfortunately, the old saying "if you don't use it, you lose it" is true when it comes to core and leg strength. Less stamina and strength in the lower half of the body is a contributing factor in the occurrence of falls.

FOUR WAYS TO PREVENT FALLS

Now that we know what can contribute to falls as we grow older, we are going to take a look at how we can be proactive and prevent falls from happening. Remember, falling is not a normal part of aging! It is avoidable with just a few preemptive steps, such as:

○ Have your eyes and feet examined. The doctor will not only look at the overall health of your eyesight, but can prescribe an updated prescription for glasses or contacts as well. Clear vision is necessary to avoid falls. Have your healthcare provider look at your feet and the shoes you normally wear, and get a recommendation for a podiatrist if necessary.

○ Get an annual checkup. Every year, get an assessment of your health from your general practitioner or healthcare provider. Talk with your doctor about any dizziness or balance issues that you have had and have them review the list of prescription medications you take to see if there are any interactions that may contribute to feelings of dizziness, drowsiness, or instability. Ask about vitamin D supplements that can improve your bone and muscle health.

○ Make your home trip-proof. Clear all the walking areas of your home from any clutter, books, or small objects that you can potentially fall over. Remove scatter rugs or tape them down securely with double-sided rug tape. Use non-slip mats in the bathroom and other areas that have tile flooring. Keep commonly used items in easy-to-reach places to avoid using step stools or ladders. Assess the lighting in your home and switch out lamps or bulbs for ones that offer clear, warm lights to help you see better.

○ Maintain a regular fitness program. Discuss with your doctor or a physical trainer how you can exercise safely and incorporate cardiovascular, strength training, flexibility, and balance exercises into a daily routine. As you gain strength, stamina, and confidence, you decrease your chances of falling and injuring yourself.

TEST YOUR BALANCE

How good is your balance? When we are young, our balance and reaction times are usually good. As we get older, however, things happen that affect our stability such as illness, injury, and medical conditions. Balance is crucial to performing everyday activities and avoiding falls, and it is easy to test our balance at home to get a general idea of how we are doing.

An important thing to remember before testing out your balance on your own is to be honest with yourself and the current condition of your health. It is normal to feel dizzy and off balance if you are ill, under the influence of alcohol or certain medications, or tired. However, if you are experiencing chronic dizziness and balance problems, you should see a doctor to get things checked out. Some warning signs that mean it's time to seek medical evaluation include:

- Periodic episodes of dizziness for no apparent reason.
- Dizziness that lasts for more than two or three days.
- Chronic dizziness that results in the inability to walk or drive safely.
- Dizziness that occurs after a fall or accident.
- Signs of confusion, slurred speech, weakness, or numbness on one side of the body.

Getting prompt diagnosis and a plan for treatment is key to avoiding future problems and increasing chances for a good outcome.

BALANCE TESTS

If you are wondering just how good your balance is, you can do this simple at-home test to get an idea. No equipment is needed.

Balance Test 1: Feet together

- Stand up tall with your feet flat on the floor and ankle bones touching each other.
- Cross your arms in front of your chest.
- Close your eyes.
- Hold this position for as long as you can.
- The standard time to hold this position is 60 seconds.

Balance Test 2: Feet tandem

- Stand up tall with your feet flat on the floor.
- Place one foot in front of the other, heel to toe.
- Close your eyes and hold this position for as long as possible.

- ○ The standard time to hold this position is 30 seconds.

Balance Test 3: One-legged stand

- ○ Stand up tall with your feet flat on the floor.
- ○ Cross your arms in front of your chest.
- ○ Bend one knee and lift that leg's foot off the floor. Don't allow this leg to touch your other one. Hold this position as long as you can.
- ○ Now, close your eyes and continue to hold this position for as long as possible.
- ○ The standard times to hold this position are:
- ○ Age 60 and younger:
- ○ Eyes open: 29 seconds
- ○ Eyes closed: 21 seconds
- ○ Age 61 and older:
- ○ Eyes open: 22 seconds
- ○ Eyes closed: 10 seconds

Balance Test 4: Alternate one-legged stand

- ○ Stand up tall with both feet flat on the ground.
- ○ Put both hands on your hips.
- ○ Raise one foot and place it against the inside of the calf of your other leg.
- ○ On your standing leg, raise your heel off the ground so you are standing on the ball of your foot.
- ○ Hold this position for as long as you can.
- ○ The standard time for this position is 25 seconds on each leg.

Balance Test 5: Stand and Reach

- ○ Stand up tall with both feet flat on the ground.
- ○ Reach forward with both arms out in front of you as far as you can.
- ○ The standard reach is 10 inches, or 25 centimeters, without losing your balance.

How did you do? If you were not able to hold these positions for their standard times, there is room for improvement in your balance. We will be working on this throughout the remainder of the book.

In this chapter, we covered a lot of information. Understanding how our body regulates our balance and equilibrium gives insight into how and why things can go awry and affect our steadiness. Fall risk factors are real and can be devastating if not addressed, so we also learned how to take preventative measures to ensure we are protected against accidental trips and slips.

What follows in the next few chapters are specific exercises to help our bodies regain and retain good balance. **Let's get started!**

Seated
Exercises

The great thing about getting older is that you don't lose all the other ages you've been.
—Madeleine L'Engle

Those who are not familiar with seated exercising may find it surprising to learn that seated exercises are not only effective, but also a low-impact and safe way to get in some cardio movement, strength training, and flexibility in a low-impact way. Regaining and maintaining your balance can also be accomplished with exercises while in a seated position. If you are recovering from a fall, stroke, or other event that has thrown off your equilibrium, starting with seated exercises is a smart way to start off, as it builds strength and balance while lessening the chance of any further falls. If you are disabled and require a wheelchair, seated exercises may be your only option, depending on the severity of your injuries. But this does not prevent you from completing these exercises and helping you regain and maintain your balance. Sitting requires balance as well and working on your stability will help you to be confident in your sitting posture and abilities to perform other tasks.

In this chapter, we will look at ten of the best seated exercises for balance. For these seated exercises, it is recommended to sit in an armless, straight-backed chair. If you need extra stability, place the chair near a table or low counter that you can place your hand upon if needed.

FORWARD PUNCH

Time per rep: 20 to 30 second   **Total time: 5 minutes**

Areas worked on: triceps, upper back, lower back, glutes, hamstrings

Directions:

1. Sit in the chair with both feet flat on the floor. Raise both arms out straight in front of you with hands clasped together.

2. Slowly lean your upper body forward while keeping your arms in front of you and as if they were reaching for something.

3. Lean as far forward as you can comfortably, hold for five seconds, then slowly return back to the original position. Repeat 10 times.

4. To level up: While leaning forward, reach down towards the floor instead of straight out in front of you. You can also try reaching diagonally.

Take Note:

This exercise mimics the everyday activity of reaching for items. Don't lean too far forward if you don't have the core strength. Only lean as far as comfortable for you.

HIP ABDUCTION SIDE KICK

Time per rep: 20 to 30 second   **Total time: 5 minutes**

Areas worked on: abdominals, quadriceps, outside of hip, inner thighs

Directions:

1. Sit in the chair with legs about hips-width apart and both feet flat on the floor.

2. Raise up the right leg and right foot off the floor. Kick the right foot out to the side, then swing it back inwards crossing over the left shin. Repeat 20 times.

3. Switch sides using the left leg and foot. Raise the left leg and foot, kicking out to the left and swinging it back in to cross over the right shin. Repeat 20 times.

4. Repeat with both legs two more times each.

Take Note:

Be sure to hold on with one or both hands to the sides of the seat or a nearby table for added stability.

HIP EXTERNAL ROTATOR STRETCH

Time per rep: 2 minute   **Total time: 6 minutes**

Areas worked on: glutes, hips, abdominals, lower back

Directions:

1. Sit in the chair with both feet on the floor. Raise the right foot and cross your legs, placing the outside of the right ankle on the left knee.

2. Slowly lean the upper body forward as far as you can. Hands can be on your crossed leg or holding onto the chair. Hold the stretch for 15 to 20 seconds, breathing normally.

3. Return to the starting position. Repeat with the left leg by crossing the left ankle on top of the right knee. Lean forward and hold for 15 to 20 seconds.

4. Repeat two more times on both sides.

5. To level up: Reach for the floor in front of you with both hands.

Take Note:

Keeping hips strong and flexible is important for balance and stability. Be sure not to lean too far forward to avoid falling out of the chair.

HIP FLEXION FOLD

Time per rep: 2 minute   **Total time: 6 minutes**

Areas worked on: abdominals, hip flexors, glutes, biceps

Directions:

1. Sit in the chair with both feet on the floor. Raise the right leg, keeping it bent. Place your hands under your right thigh and draw the leg up as far as you can without bending forward. Hold for three seconds, then lower back down. Repeat 10 times.

2. Switching legs, raise the left leg and place your hands under the left thigh. Draw the leg up and hold for three seconds before lowering back down. Repeat 10 times.

Take Note:

Pay attention that your back doesn't start rounding while doing this exercise. Keep sitting up tall and erect with good posture.

ISOMETRIC BACK EXTENSOR HOLD

Time per rep: 2 minute   **Total time: 6 minutes**

Areas worked on: abdominals, upper back, lower back

Directions:

1. Sit towards the front edge of the chair with both feet flat on the floor. Slowly lean backwards, slightly rounding your back until you can press your back onto the chair. Hold for five seconds.

2. Slowly return to the original upright position.

3. Repeat 10 times.

Take Note:

Be sure not to arch your back when you return to the upright position. For added stability, hold on to the seat with both hands.

LATERAL TRUNK FLEXION

Time per rep: 30 second   **Total time: 5 minutes**

Areas worked on: abdominals, obliques, lower back

Directions:

1. Sit in the chair with feet on the floor about hips width apart. Sitting upright with hands on the tops of the thighs, slowly tilt to the right, moving your right shoulder towards your right hip as far as you can. Hold for 10 seconds, then return to the original upright position.

2. Switching sides, now slowly tilt to the left, moving your left shoulder towards your left hip as far as you can. Hold for 10 seconds, then return to the original position.

3. Repeat on both sides two more times.

Take Note:

Mobility and flexibility in your trunk area helps with stability. Keep your neck and shoulders relaxed and avoid hunching while doing this exercise.

SEATED MARCHING

Time per rep: 3 minute   **Total time: 3 minutes**

Areas worked on: abdominals, quadriceps, hamstrings, hip flexors

Directions:

1. Sit on the chair close to the front edge, with both feet flat on the floor. Sit up tall without slouching. Hold on to the chair seat with both hands if needed.

2. Pick up the right knee and foot off the floor and lift as high as you can. Be careful not to lean back but remain upright. Put the leg down and switch legs. Lift up the left knee and foot as high as you can. Continue to alternate legs, 'marching' for about 30 seconds.

3. Rest for 30 seconds, then repeat once more.

Take Note:

Being able to lift your leg and foot high enough to clear curbs and stairs without losing your balance is an important skill. Don't lean back or let your back start to round as you bring your legs up. Remain sitting up tall and erect.

SIT-TO-STAND

Time per rep: 30 second

Total time: 5 minutes

Areas worked on: abdominals, back, glutes, quadriceps, hamstrings

Directions:

1. Sit in a chair with your feet flat on the floor and about hips-width apart. Feet should be slightly behind the knees for leverage.

2. Slowly stand up and remain standing for 10 seconds as you regain balance. Use your hands and arms if needed. Return to a seated position.

3. Repeat 10 times.

4. To level up: Hold a five pound weight between your hands while you do this exercise for added resistance.

Take Note:

Going from a sitting to standing position is a daily skill that is needed. Ensure that the chair you use in this exercise is sturdy and will not move as you sit, stand, and return to sit.

TOE RAISES

Time per rep: 3 minute   **Total time: 3 minutes**

Areas worked on: acalves, feet

Directions:

1. Sit in a chair with your feet flat on the floor. Place your hands on the tops of your thighs.

2. Slowly raise your toes off the floor. You may notice your upper body wanting to lean back, but stay upright and slightly lean forward if you need to. Hold for 10 seconds, then lower toes back down.

3. Repeat 10 times.

4. To level up: Alternate between raising toes and raising heels.

Take Note:

Calf muscle strength is important for ankle stability. If your calf muscles start to burn, take a rest between repetitions.

TRUNK CIRCLES

Time per rep: 15 second   **Total time: 2 minute 30 second**

Areas worked on: abdominals, obliques, lower back

Directions:

1. Sit in a chair with your feet flat on the floor and hips-width apart. Place your hands on top of your thighs.

2. Keep the lower body stationery while you move your shoulders and torso forward, right, back, and left in a clockwise motion. Make 10 big circles. Switch directions and move shoulders and torso forward, left, back, and right in a counter-clockwise motion for 10 circles.

3. Repeat two more times in each direction.

4. To level up: Hold your arms straight out from your sides while doing the exercise.

Take Note:

This exercise helps train the body in weight shifts and directional changes. Keep your eyes focused on a stationary object straight in front of you for added balance.

Standing Exercises

You can't help getting older, but you don't have to get old.

—*George Burns*

Balance exercises done while standing help improve muscle strength while working on balance. Holding on to the back of a chair, countertop, or railing allows for extra stability while you work on your balance. In this chapter, we look at the 10 best balance exercises to do from a standing position. These standing exercises are dynamic ways to build your balance to accomplish everyday activities and tasks, such as going up and down stairs, turning, stepping in narrow spaces, and reaching for items.

Standing exercises are not only good for strengthening the larger muscles in your legs, like the hamstrings, quadriceps, and calves, it is also key to making the smaller muscles like those in your ankles and feet stronger. Ankle strength and steadiness is an important factor in balance. The loss of ankle strength can lead to challenges in standing, walking, turning around, and even driving.

If you are recovering from an injury or just need extra help, enlist someone to help you as a spotter who will catch you if you lose your balance. As you get stronger and want to make these exercises more challenging, you can adjust your hold. Start off using two hands on a chair or countertop, then level up to using only one hand. When you find that using one hand is easy, you can then try doing the exercises with only one finger on a chair for balance or maybe even without holding on at all. Go slowly and give yourself time to progress.

3-WAY HIP KICK

Time per rep: 30 second   **Total time: 5 minutes**

Areas worked on: abdominals, hips

Directions:

1. Stand up tall with your feet about hips-width apart. Place hands on the back of a chair or on a countertop.

2. Extend your right foot and point it out in front of you. Return to the original position. Now extend the right foot out to the right side and then return. Finally, extend the right foot to the back and then return. If the floor was a clock, your right foot would point towards the 12, the 3, and the 6 o'clock positions.

3. Switch legs and now extend the left foot to the front, the left, and the back. Your right foot would point towards the 12, the 9, and the 6 o'clock positions.

4. Repeat 10 times on each leg.

Take Note:

Strength in the hip muscles are important for walking, changing direction, and going up and down stairs. Take care not to arch your lower back while completing this exercise.

FOOT TAPS

Time per rep: 30 second   **Total time: 5 minutes**

Areas worked on: abdominals, hip flexor, quadriceps, calves

Directions:

1. Place a step stool, thick book, or small cone next to a chair or countertop.

2. Stand up tall with your feet hips-width apart. Hold on to the chair or countertop with both hands.

3. Lift your right foot and tap the step, book, or cone with your toes or ball of the foot. Return your foot to the starting position. Repeat 10 times.

4. Switch legs and lift your left foot and tap the step. Return to the starting position and then repeat 10 times.

5. Repeat each leg two more times.

Take Note:

This exercise mimics going up a flight of stairs. Be sure to raise your foot before tapping to avoid stumbling.

HEEL RAISES

Time per rep: 30 second   **Total time: 5 minutes**

Areas worked on: calves, ankles, feet

Directions:

1. Stand up tall with your feet hips-width apart. Use both hands to hold on to the back of a chair or countertop.

2. Slowly lift your heels off the ground and feel your weight shift into the front towards your toes. You can use your hands for support, but be sure not to lean your body weight onto them. Lower the heels to the ground. Repeat 10 times.

3. Rest for 15 seconds, then repeat exercise once more.

4. To level up: Use only one hand or one finger on the counter for stability. When comfortable with the exercise, try doing it without the help of any hands.

Take Note:

Calf muscles help with ankle stability and overall balance. Be sure you keep good posture while doing this exercise and not lean over onto the counter.

LATERAL STEPPING

Time per rep: 1 minute **Total time: 3 minutes**

Areas worked on: abdominals, lower back, glutes, quadriceps, hamstrings, calves

Directions:

1. Stand up tall with your feet together. Hold on to the back of a chair or countertop.

2. Step your right foot out to the side, just past your shoulder, and slightly bend your knee as you put weight on the right foot. Return the foot to the original position. Repeat 10 times.

3. Switch legs and now step your left foot out to the side just past your shoulder. Return the foot to the starting position and repeat 10 times.

4. Repeat exercise two more times on each leg.

5. To level up: Once you are comfortable doing this exercise, try doing it without holding on with your hands.

Take Note:

Lateral exercises like this improve coordination in tight spaces. Concentrate on picking up your foot before stepping to avoid tripping. Be sure all loose rugs or other objects are away from the exercise area.

MINI LUNGES

Time per rep: 45 second   **Total time: 2 minutes**

Areas worked on: abdominals, glutes, quadriceps, hamstrings, calves, ankles

Directions:

1. Stand up tall with feet hips-width apart. Hold on to the back of a chair or countertop.

2. Step your right foot forward and bend your right knee slightly. This is not a deep lunge and should not be painful in any way. Bring your foot back to the starting position. Repeat 10 times.

3. Switch legs and step forward with your left foot, bending the left knee slightly. Bring the foot back to the starting position, then repeat 10 times.

4. Repeat exercise two more times on each leg.

5. To level up: When you are comfortable, use only one finger on the chair for stability.

Take Note:

This exercise mimics forward stepping while strengthening the entire leg. Take care to not go too deep in the lunge to avoid straining muscles.

NARROW STANCE REACH

Time per rep: 1 minute   **Total time: 3 minutes**

Areas worked on: shoulders, upper back, lower back, glutes, hamstrings

Directions:

1. Stand up tall with feet fairly close together. With your left hand holding on to the back of a chair or countertop, reach forward with the right hand extending as far as it is comfortable. Bring the right hand back to the starting position. Repeat the right hand reaching for 10 times.

2. Switch arms by holding on to the chair with the right hand. Reach forward with the left hand and extend as far as you can. Bring the hand back and repeat the left hand reaching for 10 times.

3. Repeat exercise two more times on each arm.

4. To level up: As you get stronger, you can try reaching with both hands at the same time. You can also reach out to the sides for a directional change.

Take Note:

Reaching for items at the back of a cabinet or shelf without losing your balance is an everyday skill. Be sure to keep both feet on the ground to maintain a stable base while reaching.

SINGLE LEG STANCE

Time per rep: 2 minute   **Total time: 6 minutes**

Areas worked on: abdominals, quadriceps, hamstrings, calves, ankles

Directions:

1. Stand up tall with feet about hips-width apart. Hold on to the chair or countertop with both hands.

2. Lift the right foot off the floor, continuing to stand tall without leaning too much on the standing leg. Hold for 10 seconds, then lower the right foot back down. Repeat 10 times.

3. Switch legs and lift the left foot off the floor, standing tall, and holding for 10 seconds. Lower the foot and repeat 10 times.

Take Note:

We stand on a single leg more than we realize. Everytime you take a step, go up and down stairs, or get into a bathtub, you spend time on one leg. As you progress, do this exercise without holding onto anything with your hands.

SQUATS

Time per rep: 30 second   **Total time: 1 minute**

Areas worked on: abdominals, lower back, glutes, quadriceps, hamstrings, calves

Directions:

1. Stand up tall with your feet hips-width apart. Place your hands on a chair or countertop for stability.

2. Bend both knees and squat, as if you were going to sit down in a chair. Return to a standing position. Repeat 10 times.

3. Rest for 15 seconds, then repeat the exercise 10 more times.

4. To level up: Use only one hand for stability while doing this exercise.

Take Note:

Squatting is an essential skill for sitting in a chair or getting into a car. If you are unsure of your ability to come back up from a squat, you can position a sturdy chair behind you that will catch you if you cannot rise from the squat.

STANDING MARCHES

Time per rep: 5 minute   **Total time: 5 minutes**

Areas worked on: abdominals, glutes, quadriceps, hamstrings, hip flexors

Directions:

1. Stand up tall with your feet hips-width apart. Hold onto a countertop or back of a chair with either your right or left hand.

2. Bend your right leg and raise your right foot as high as you can while remaining upright. Return the right foot to the floor.

3. Bend your left leg and raise your left foot as high as you can, then return it to the floor.

4. Continue 'marching' by lifting one foot and then the other, alternating until you have done it 20 times.

5. Rest if needed, then do the exercise one more time.

Take Note:

This exercise helps with single leg balance and the strength of your hips. Be sure to keep good posture and stand up tall while doing this exercise. Avoid rounding your back or hunching forward.

TANDEM STANCE

Time per rep: 30 second   **Total time: 5 minutes**

Areas worked on: aabdominals, lower back, hips

Directions:

1. Stand up tall and hold on to a countertop or the back of a chair with both hands or one hand.

2. Move the right foot and place it directly in front of the left one. Right heel should be in front of the left toes. In this narrow stance, hold the position for 1o seconds.

3. Switch feet by moving the left foot and putting it in front of the right. The left heel should be in front of the right toes. Hold for 10 seconds.

4. Repeat 10 times.

Take Note:

Because this exercise causes you to have a narrower base of support, you may feel off balance quickly. Your core muscles will help your stability, so tighten your abs and glutes while doing this exercise.

Walking
Exercises

I love wood. I love its permanence, its way of changing hue over the years, its way of expanding and contracting, of moving or aging and growing better and more beautiful with time.

—David Linley

Walking requires balance. Your center of gravity changes each time you take a step, so as you walk, your body is constantly working to maintain equilibrium to keep you upright. Working on your balance as you walk is a good way to incorporate movement into your balance exercises. Training your body in this way helps it to respond to shifts in balance while you are moving and helps to build stability.

It is important to maintain good posture while you are walking. You should be standing straight with your shoulders back and relaxed, with your hands down by your sides. Keep your stomach pulled in and your core tight to prevent any leaning forward or backwards, which can put a strain on your back. It's also good to keep your chin parallel to the ground and your gaze looking ahead of you to reduce any pressure on your neck as well as being able to spot what's ahead on your path. Regularly check your posture at intervals during your walk and make adjustments in it to build good posture habits. Over time, your body will gravitate towards keeping a good alignment and posture.

In this chapter, we look at the ten easy ways to incorporate balance exercises while walking across a room. You can also do these while on your daily walks in your neighborhood or on a treadmill. If you are recovering from injury or have trouble walking, be sure to have a companion that can walk with you and assist you if needed.

BACKWARD WALKING

Time per rep: 1 minute 30 second   **Total time: 3 minutes**

Areas worked on: abdominals, glutes, hips, quadriceps, hamstrings, calves, ankles

Directions:

1. This exercise is best done with a partner that can alert you to any tripping hazards. Be sure to walk on a flat, level area. If you are on a sidewalk, make sure you are away from traffic and other pedestrians. This can also be done on a treadmill.

2. To start, walk forward 10 steps. Turn around and continue to walk in the same direction but facing backwards. Walk slowly for 10 steps. Turn around again and continue to walk 10 steps forward.

3. Repeat for 2 minutes, alternating between walking 10 steps facing forward and 10 steps facing backward all while walking in one direction.

4. To level up: Once you are comfortable walking backwards, walk for 20 steps instead of 10 steps.

Take Note:

This exercise helps your core muscles respond to directional changes as well as working your leg muscles in different ways. Take care not to walk too quickly when walking backwards to avoid falling.

BALANCE WALKING

Time per rep: 30 second   **Total time: 3 minutes**

Areas worked on: shoulders, abdominals, hip flexors, glutes, hamstrings, ankles

Directions:

1. Standing up tall, bring your arms up and out straight from the sides of your body to about shoulder height.

2. Take one step forward with your right foot and as you bring your left foot from behind you to take the next step, bend your left knee and lift your left foot up. Pause for 1 second before following through with the rest of the step forward with your left foot.

3. Do the same thing now with your right foot. As you bring your right leg forward for the next step, bend your right knee and lift the right foot, holding it up for 1 second before completing the step. Repeat for 20 steps.

4. Rest for a few seconds, then repeat exercise once more.

Take Note:

This exercise is similar to the standing marches but with forward movement. The ankle muscles are being strengthened as they help your body stabilize. If you need support, have a partner hold one of your hands.

BALL TOSS

Time per rep: 1 minute 30 second   **Total time: 3 minutes**

Areas worked on: hands, forearms, glutes, hip flexors, hamstrings, calves

Directions:

1. Bring a small squishy ball with you on your walk. As you walk forward, squish the ball in your right hand as you walk 10 steps forward.

2. Toss the ball to your left hand and squish the ball in your left hand as you continue walking for another 10 steps.

3. Repeat two more times in each hand.

Take Note:

By having to multitask, your body will adjust its balance and coordination. Be sure you keep your eyes focused on where you are walking to avoid tripping.

CURB WALKING

Time per rep: 30 second   **Total time: 1 minute**

Areas worked on: abdominals, hips, glutes, inner thighs, hamstrings, calves

Directions:

1. Try walking in a straight line on a slightly raised surface like a two-by-four length of wood or a curb. If you are outside, be sure that you are walking somewhere away from traffic and with a friend. You can place your hand on their shoulder for support or hold their arm.

2. If you are unsure about walking on something as tall as a curb, try walking in a straight line, heel-to-toe, on a flat path.

Take Note:

This exercise requires a narrower stance, which gives you a smaller base of stability. Walk slow and heel-to-toe to avoid falling off the curb.

DYNAMIC WALKING

Time per rep: 30 second   **Total time: 30 second**

Areas worked on: neck, abdominals, hip flexors, glutes, hamstrings, calves

Directions:

1. Do this first in your living room or backyard until you get used to it. Starting at one end of your room or yard, walk slowly towards the opposite side.

2. While continuing to walk straight, slowly turn your head to the right and then to the left while walking. Continue turning your head to the right and left slowly until you reach the other side of the room.

3. Repeat 10 times.

4. To level up: As you get more confident, you can incorporate this into your walks outside at the park or in your neighborhood.

Take Note:

This exercise requires a shift in your focus each time you turn your head. Be sure to turn your head slowly to avoid dizziness. If you feel dizzy at any time, stop.

GRAPEVINE

Time per rep: 30 second   **Total time: 1 minute**

Areas worked on: abdominals, hips, inner thighs, quadriceps, calves

Directions:

1. You can hold onto a countertop as you do this exercise or have a partner hold on to your hands if you feel unsteady.

2. Start by standing up tall with your feet together. Cross your right foot over your left and step down. Uncross by bringing your left foot back and place it next to your right so both feet are together normally. Continue crossing your right foot over your left for 10 steps or until you reach the other end of the countertop.

3. Go back in the other direction by now crossing your left foot behind your right and stepping to the right. Uncross by bringing your right foot up and placing it next to your left. Continue crossing your left foot behind as you travel to the right for 10 steps or reach the end of the counter.

4. Repeat five times.

5. To level up: If you get very comfortable with this exercise, you can make it more challenging by alternating crossing in front and crossing behind every other step.

Take Note:

At first you may find yourself looking down at your feet, but remember to look up and see where you are going. Try to keep your head up.

HEEL-TO-TOE

Time per rep: 1 minute   **Total time: 5 minute**

Areas worked on: abdominals, hips, inner thighs, quadriceps, hamstrings, calves

Directions:

1. You can hold onto a countertop as you do this exercise or have a partner hold on to your hands if you feel unsteady.

2. Stand up tall and put your right foot directly in front of your left. Walk heel-to-toe as if you were walking on a tightrope. Continue walking heel-to-toe for 15 steps or until you reach the other end of the counter or opposite side of the room.

3. Repeat five times.

4. To level up: To make this more challenging, you can place masking tape or blue painters tape in a straight line on your floor. Practice walking on the line, without holding onto anything.

Take Note:

This exercise requires a narrower stance and will challenge your balance because of a smaller base of support. You can raise your arms away from your sides to help with stability if you are not holding onto anything.

SIDE STEPS

Time per rep: 1 minute   **Total time: 5 minute**

Areas worked on: abdominals, hip abductors, quadriceps, glutes, calves

Directions:

1. Practice this first in your living room or backyard until you are confident in your ability. Standing up tall, step to the right with your right foot and bring your left foot to meet your right. Continue sidestepping to the right 10 times.

2. Change direction and now step to the left with your left foot. Bring your right foot to meet your left and continue sidestepping to the left 10 times.

3. Repeat five times.

4. To level up: Once you are self-assured in this move, you can practice this on your walks outside. Turn sideways while walking and side step for 10 steps in one direction before switching to the other side. Remember to always keep your head facing the direction you are moving.

Take Note:

Sidestepping is an everyday skill that you use at home, in stores, and anywhere there are people around. Avoid looking down at your feet. Instead look straight ahead or in the direction you are moving.

HEEL-TO-TOE

Heel-to-Toe

Time per rep: 30 second   **Total time: 1 minutes 30 second**

Areas worked on: abdominals, hip flexors, calves

Directions:

1. Be sure to warm up your legs and feet by walking normally for five minutes before starting this exercise. You can hold onto a countertop or enlist the help of a friend if you need added support.

2. Walk slowly forward on your heels with your toes lifted off the ground. Walk for 10 steps.

3. Walk forward normally for 10 steps.

4. Now, slowly walk on your toes with your heels lifted off the ground. Walk for 10 steps.

5. Repeat two times.

Take Note:

If your calves or feet are starting to cramp, take a break, and do only half the steps. Increase the amount of steps only when you are comfortable.

ZIGZAG WALKING

Time per rep: 1 minute   **Total time: 5 minute**

Areas worked on: abdominals, hips, quadriceps, hamstrings, calves

Directions:

1. This exercise requires directional shifts to increase your balance while walking. You can set up two cones six feet apart and walk in a figure eight pattern around the cones. Repeat five times.

2. Alternatively, you can walk in a zigzag pattern on a path or sidewalk. Walk forward at an angle towards the right side of the path, then walk forward towards the left side of the path. Zigzag back and forth across the path several times.

Take Note:

Because walking in a serpentine pattern means a change in directions, your balance will be challenged. Keep your core muscles engaged as you walk.

Core
Exercises

Aging has a wonderful beauty and we should have respect for that.
—Eartha Kitt

Our core is the area from the lower ribs all the way down the trunk of the body to the buttocks. The core muscles are important for balance and stabilization in our bodies. These muscles include the muscles in the stomach and belly area, the obliques on the side of the body, and the back muscles. They are important in helping us complete everyday tasks such as getting out of bed, sitting, standing, and bending over. Providing stability to the back, arms, and legs, the core muscles need regular exercise to remain strong. When these muscles are exercised, they also help support a healthy back and minimize back pain.

There was a time when core exercises consisted mainly of sit-ups and crunches. These used to be the gold standard to not only getting a trim midsection but also a strong core. But as we get older, these exercises can cause problems with our aging necks and backs. Pulling on your neck and pushing your spine against a hard surface, even if it is lightly padded, is hard on your entire back. Degenerative disc disease, back problems, and arthritis can also make sit-ups and crunches painful and difficult. Additionally, those exercises only work a few stomach muscles and not the rest of the core. Sit-ups and crunches mainly target the hip flexors, which are the muscles that run along the lower back to the thighs. Overworking the hip flexors can cause them to become overly strong or too tight, resulting in lower back pain and discomfort.

In this chapter, we will learn ten of the best exercises to strengthen your core and how to exercise a variety of core muscles. When we train the entire set of core muscles, instead of just a few muscles in isolation, we are having those muscles work together like they do in our everyday movements.

BRIDGE

Time per rep: 30 second   **Total time: 5 minute**

Areas worked on: lower back, glutes, hamstrings, calves

Directions:

1. Lie on your back facing up on the floor or a padded mat. Bend your knees and keep your feet flat on the floor about hips-width apart. Arms should be on the floor by your sides.

2. Tighten up your buttocks. Lift your hips off the floor so that your lower back and mid back are also off the floor. Your shoulders, hips, and knees should form a straight line. Hold for 10 seconds, then gently lower to the floor.

3. Repeat 10 times.

Take Note:

The closer your feet are to your glutes, the harder it will be to lift your hips off the floor, so adjust the distance accordingly. Remember to lower back down to the floor with control.

FOREARM PLANK

Time per rep: 30 second   **Total time: 5 minute**

Areas worked on: shoulders, upper back, abdominals

Directions:

1. Facing the ground or a mat on the floor, lie face down with your forearms on the ground. Be sure that your elbows are directly under your shoulders and that your back is not arching.

2. Tighten your core and press into your forearms and toes to lift your body off the floor. Press your belly button in towards your spine and squeeze your buttocks to help stabilize your body and keep it in a straight line. Hold for 20 seconds. Slowly lower to the floor.

3. Repeat five times.

4. 4To level up: Support your body on your hands instead of your forearms. Hands should be flat on the floor directly under the shoulders.

Take Note:

Do not allow your hips to sag, causing a sway in the lower back. Your body should be in a straight diagonal line from your shoulders to feet.

MODIFIED PLANK

Time per rep: 30 second   **Total time: 5 minute**

Areas worked on: shoulders, upper back, abdominals

Directions:

1. Start with your hands and knees on the floor and your gaze facing down.

2. Lower your forearms down to the floor and support your upper body on them. Your knees, hips, and shoulders should form a straight line like in a regular plank. Hold the position for 30 seconds. Slowly lower to the ground.

3. Repeat five times.

Take Note:

This is the modified version of the forearm plank for those who are still building core strength. If you have any knee issues, you may want to put a folded towel or other padding under your knees.

OPPOSITE ARM AND LEG RAISE

Time per rep: 30 second   **Total time: 5 minute**

Areas worked on: shoulders, upper back, lower back, glutes, hamstrings

Directions:

1. Start with your hands and knees on the floor and your gaze facing down. Keep your neck neutral and in line with your spine.

2. Straighten your right leg and extend your right foot behind you, toes pointing down to the ground. Try to bring your leg up so it is parallel to the floor. If you can, raise the opposite arm, your left arm, and extend it out in front of you while still looking down. Hold the position for 10 seconds, then slowly lower your arm and leg back down to the ground. Repeat five times.

3. Switch sides by now straightening your left leg and foot out behind you. Raise your right arm and extend it out in front of you. Hold the position for 10 seconds, then slowly lower back to the ground. Repeat on this side five times.

4. Repeat the exercise on both sides twice more.

Take Note:

If keeping your arm up is too challenging, you can hold on to something sturdy in front of you, like a chair or table leg to help with balance.

SEATED FORWARD ROLL UP

Time per rep: 30 second   **Total time: 2 minute 30 second**

Areas worked on: abdominals

Directions:

1. Sit up tall in a chair towards the front edge of the seat. Extend your legs straight out in front of you with your feet on the floor and flexed toward you.

2. Extend your arms out in front of you and slowly lower your chin towards your chest. Roll your back and chest forward as you reach your hands towards your feet. Engage your abdominal muscles to hold you steady.

3. Once you have reached your hands as far as you can, slowly roll back up to the starting position.

4. Repeat 10 times.

Take Note:

Remember to go slowly and not use momentum in this exercise.

SEATED HALF ROLL-BACKS

Time per rep: 30 second   **Total time: 1 minute**

Areas worked on: abdominals, upper back, lower back

Directions:

1. Sit up tall in a chair towards the front edge of the seat. Keep your knees bent and feet flat on the floor.

2. Lift your arms out in front of you so they form a circle with your fingertips touching. Round your back and tighten your abdominal muscles as you bring your chin to your chest. Hold the position for 10 seconds, then slowly roll up and return to the starting position.

3. Repeat 10 times.

Take Note:

Be sure to start with an upright posture before rounding and return to the same upright position. Don't slouch or lean back into the chair.

SEATED LEG LIFTS

Time per rep: 30 second   **Total time: 2 minute 30 second**

Areas worked on: abdominals, hip flexors, quadriceps

Directions:

1. Sit up tall in a chair with your knees bent and feet flat on the floor. Hands can be on the tops of your thighs or holding on the sides of the seat.

2. Slowly straighten the right leg and lift the right foot off the floor. Try to bring the right leg as high as you can but don't let your back start to round. Keep your back upright and straight. Hold your leg up for five seconds, then slowly lower to the starting position.

3. Switch legs by straightening your left leg and lifting the left foot off the floor. Bring it up as high as you can and hold for five seconds. Slowly lower to the starting position.

4. Repeat each leg 10 times.

5. To level up: Once you are stronger, try doing the exercise with your arms straight out in front of you.

Take Note:

Don't let your back become round or collapse as you lift your leg.

SEATED LEG TAPS

Time per rep: 30 second   **Total time: 5 minute**

Areas worked on: abdominals, hip flexors, quadriceps

Directions:

1. Sit up tall in a chair with your knees bent and feet flat on the floor. Place your hands on the sides of the seat for support.

2. Tighten your abdominal muscles and straighten both legs out in front of you, lifting both feet off the floor. Try to bring the legs parallel to the floor. Slowly lower your right foot and tap the floor. Bring it back up. Slowly lower your left foot and tap the floor. Bring it back up.

3. Continue alternating tapping the right foot and then the left.

4. Repeat 10 times.

5. To level up: To make it more challenging, raise and lower both feet at the same time.

Take Note:

If you need to take a break, lower both feet to the floor for a quick rest before repeating the exercise.

SEATED SIDE BENDS

Time per rep: 30 second   **Total time: 5 minute**

Areas worked on: abdominals, obliques

Directions:

1. Sit up tall in a chair with your knees bent and feet flat on the floor. Arms should be hanging at your sides.

2. Bend and raise your right arm, placing your right hand gently on the side of your head while looking straight ahead. Bend at the waist and lean your upper body to the left. Extend your left hand down towards the floor as far as you can as you continue looking straight ahead. Slowly come back up to the starting position. Repeat 10 times.

3. Switch sides and raise your left arm, placing your left hand on the side of your head. Extend your right hand down towards the floor as you bend at the waist and lean to the right. Remember to keep looking straight ahead. Come back up to the starting position. Repeat 1o times.

4. Rest, then repeat the exercise one more time on both sides.

5. To level up: Straighten your bent arm above your head as you lean your body to the side.

Take Note:

Pay attention to your neck and shoulders. Don't hunch up. Keep your shoulders down and away from your ears.

SUPERMAN

Time per rep: 30 second   **Total time: 5 minute**

Areas worked on: abdominals, upper back, lower back, hip flexors, glutes

Directions:

1. Lie on the floor or a padded mat, facing down. Extend your arms out straight over your head and legs out straight out behind you. Your body should form a straight line.

2. Tighten the abdominal muscles as you lift your hands and feet off the floor. Keep your neck neutral and gaze looking at the floor. Hold the lifted position for 10 seconds, then slowly lower back down to the ground.

3. Repeat 10 times.

Take Note:

To avoid straining your neck, keep your gaze down and look at the floor.

Vestibular Exercises

Nothing matters more than your health. Healthy living is priceless. What millionaire wouldn't pay dearly for an extra 10 or 20 years of healthy aging?
—Peter Diamandis

Our brains interpret the information that it receives from our eyes, ears, and other senses. If there is an injury or something happens to disrupt the way the brain receives this input, that can result in equilibrium and balance problems. The resulting dizziness can make day to day activities like walking, turning, and driving more challenging. Retraining the brain with exercises that induce dizziness in a controlled manner and the means to overcome it helps build up strength and tolerance in the vestibular system. If you are having dizziness, it is important to first visit your doctor to get it checked out and identify the root cause of it.

Vestibular exercises can help us regain any balance that has been lost. These exercises train the eyes and brain to interpret the information being received and, initially, they may cause some dizziness. To avoid any injury or falls, do these exercises while seated.

EYES SIDE-TO-SIDE

Time per rep: 30 second   **Total time: 1 minute**

Areas worked on: ocular muscles

Directions:

1. Sit up tall in a chair with your knees bent and feet flat on the floor. Hold on to the seat or to a tabletop with one hand.

2. Raise the other arm out in front of you. Focus your eyes on your index finger. Move your finger to the right of you and to the left and follow your finger, moving only your eyes. Keep your head still while your eyes move. Move your finger back and forth 10 to 20 times.

3. Rest for a few seconds and repeat once more.

Take Note:

If you feel yourself getting dizzy, stop and close your eyes for a moment.

EYES UP AND DOWN

Time per rep: 30 second   **Total time: 1 minute**

Areas worked on: ocular muscles

Directions:

1. Sit up tall in a chair with your knees bent and feet flat on the floor. Hold on to the seat or to a tabletop with one hand.

2. Raise the other arm out in front of you. Focus your eyes on your index finger. Move your finger up towards the ceiling then down towards the floor. Keeping your head still, follow your finger with only your eyes. Move your finger up and down 10 to 20 times.

Take Note:

Keep your head still and level, with your chin parallel to the floor. Only your eyes should be moving.

GAZE STABILIZATION SITTING

Time per rep: 30 second   **Total time: 1 minute**

Areas worked on: ocular muscles, neck

Directions:

1. Sit up tall in a chair with your knees bent and feet flat on the floor. Hold on to the seat or to a tabletop with one or both hands.

2. Focus your eyes on an object or picture three to ten feet away from you. Preferably this object or picture will have a blank, not patterned wall behind it. While keeping your eyes focused on the object, turn your head to the right, then to the left. Keep moving your head from side to side while remaining focused on the object. Turn side to side 20 to 30 times.

Take Note:

Take care to hold on to the seat or tabletop to avoid potential falling.

GAZE STABILIZATION STANDING

Time per rep: 30 second   **Total time: 1 minute**

Areas worked on: ocular muscles

Directions:

1. Stand up tall with both hands on the back of a chair or on a countertop.

2. Focus your eyes on an object or picture three to ten feet away from you. Preferably this object or picture will have a blank, not patterned wall behind it. While keeping your eyes focused on the object, move your head up, then down. Keep moving your head up and down while remaining focused on the object. Move your head up and down 20 to 30 times.

Take Note:

To avoid falling, ensure that the chair you are holding on to is sturdy.

HEAD AND EYES OPPOSITE DIRECTION

Time per rep: 30 second   **Total time: 1 minute**

Areas worked on: ocular muscles, neck

Directions:

1. Sit up tall in a chair with your knees bent and feet flat on the floor. Hold on to the seat or to a tabletop with one hand.

2. In the other hand, hold a pencil or other small object out in front of you. While keeping your eyes focused on the pencil, move the pencil to the right as you move your head to the left. Reverse the motion by moving the pencil to the left as you move your head to the right and keep focusing on the pencil with your eyes. Repeat 20 times.

3. Rest and repeat exercise once more.

4. To level up: As you get better at this exercise, you can do it standing up.

Take Note:

Do this exercise slowly and avoid hunching up your shoulders.

HEAD AND EYES SAME DIRECTION

Time per rep: 30 second

Total time: 1 minute

Areas worked on: ocular muscles

Directions:

1. Sit up tall in a chair with your knees bent and feet flat on the floor. Hold on to the seat or to a tabletop with one hand.

2. In the other hand, hold a pencil or other small object out in front of you. While keeping your eyes focused on the pencil, move it to the right and allow your head and eyes to follow it. Reverse the motion and move the pencil to the left, moving your head and eyes along with it.

3. You can change direction and move the object up and down, allowing your head and eyes to follow. Repeat 20 times.

4. Rest and repeat once more.

5. To level up: Once you are comfortable with the exercise, try doing it standing up.

Take Note:

Keep your shoulders and upper body fairly stationary. Avoid leaning over as you move the object up and down.

HEAD BEND

Time per rep: 30 second   **Total time: 1 minute**

Areas worked on: ocular muscles, neck

Directions:

1. Sit up tall in a chair with your knees bent and feet flat on the floor. Hold on to the seat or to a tabletop with one or both hands.

2. Bend your neck and head to look down at the floor, then bring them up to look at the ceiling. Let your eyes lead your head as you continue to look down and then up 10 times.

3. Rest and repeat two times.

4. To level up: Do the exercise while standing.

Take Note:

Keep your posture tall and upright while doing the exercise. Don't lean forward or backwards.

HEAD TURN

Time per rep: 30 second   **Total time: 1 minute**

Areas worked on: ocular muscles

Directions:

1. Sit up tall in a chair with your knees bent and feet flat on the floor. Hold on to the seat or to a tabletop with one or both hands.

2. Turn your neck and head to the right as you look to the right with your eyes. Then turn your neck and head to the left as you look left. Let your eyes lead your head as you continue to look right and left, as if you were watching a tennis match, for 10 times.

3. Rest and repeat two times.

4. To level up: Stand up tall and hold on to a chair while doing the exercise.

Take Note:

Only turn your eyes and your head, not your whole body.

SHOULDER TURNS

Time per rep: 30 second   **Total time: 1 minute**

Areas worked on: abdominals, obliques, upper back, lower back

Directions:

1. Sit up tall in a chair with your knees bent and feet flat on the floor. Hold on to the seat with one or both hands.

2. Rotate your head and upper body as you turn to the right, then to the left, keeping your eyes open. Repeat 20 times.

3. Do the exercise again, but this time with your eyes closed as you turn to the right and left. Repeat 20 times.

4. Rest and repeat two more times.

5. To level up: If you are comfortable, do this exercise while standing and holding onto a chair or countertop.

Take Note:

It may be helpful to have a partner to help you while you do this with your eyes closed to ensure you don't fall.

SMOOTH PURSUITS

Time per rep: 1 minute **Total time: 3 minute**

Areas worked on: ocular muscles

Directions:

1. Sit up tall in a chair with your knees bent and feet flat on the floor. Hold on to the seat or to a tabletop with one hand.

2. Hold a pencil or small object in the other hand. Keeping your head still, move the pencil in a diagonal fashion while your eyes follow the moving object. Move the object from the lower left to upper right and vice versa, or in a zigzag pattern. Repeat 20 times.

3. Rest and repeat two times.

Take Note:

Remember to keep your head still and move your eyes only.

Vestibular Exercises

One day you will look back and see that all along you were blooming.
—Morgan Harper Nichols

We have looked at 50 exercises that can help strengthen your body and brain to regain and maintain balance. That number of exercises may seem overwhelming to you, especially if you don't have a plan to incorporate them into your daily schedule. It is important to have a plan to utilize the information here so that each day, you can just "plug and play" your exercise routine.

Some options for exercise routines include:

- One a day. Methodically working through each exercise on your own schedule. Do one exercise a day until you work through all 50 exercises.

- Chapter focused. Another alternative is to work through the exercises chapter-by-chapter. For instance, if you did one move a day from the chapter on seated exercises, you would complete them all in ten days. If you did two moves a day, you would complete the chapter in five days.

- Routines. Finally, you can follow the carefully crafted routines that are presented in this chapter. There is a month's worth of exercise plans. The routines are weekly, five days a week. The schedules include a week focused on core moves, a week concentrating on leg strength, a week devoted to brain training, and, finally, a week of walking and movement.

CORE FOCUS WEEK

The concentration of this weekly routine is core strength and foundational seated exercises. As we learned in an earlier chapter, the core muscles include the abdominal, back, and glute muscles. These muscles provide needed stabilization for your body, arms, and legs to move about and function. Strong core muscles also help alleviate back pain while building balance.

Day 1

- Bridge (Ch. 5)
- Modified Plank (Ch. 5)
- Superman (Ch. 5)
- Hip External Rotator Stretch (Ch. 2)

Day 2

- Seated Forward Roll Up (Ch. 5)
- Seated Side Bend (Ch. 5)
- Seated Marching (Ch. 2)
- Isometric Back Extensor (Ch. 2)

Day 3

- Forearm Plank (Ch. 5)
- Opposite Arm and Leg Raise (Ch. 5)
- Lateral Trunk Flexion (Ch. 2)
- Forward Punch (Ch. 2)

Day 4

- Seated Half Roll-Backs (Ch. 5)
- Seated Leg Lifts (Ch. 5)
- Seated Leg Taps (Ch. 5)
- Hip Abduction Side Kicks (Ch. 2)

Day 5

- Hip Flexion (Ch. 2)
- Toe Raises (Ch. 2)
- Sit-to-Stand (Ch. 2)
- Trunk Circles (Ch. 2)

LEG STRENGTH WEEK

The objective of this week's exercises is to build strength and balance in the lower half of the body, particularly the legs. Falls, strokes, and accidents can result in one leg being weaker than the other, causing imbalances over time. The exercises this week will concentrate on strengthening both legs and the lower body while maintaining equilibrium.

Day 1

- Seated Marching (Ch. 2)
- Hip External Rotator Stretch (Ch. 2)
- Single Leg Stance (Ch. 3)
- Foot Taps (Ch. 3)

Day 2

- Hip Flexion Fold (Ch. 2)
- Sit-to-Stand (Ch. 2)
- Standing Marches (Ch. 3)
- Squats (Ch. 3)

Day 3

- Hip Abduction Side Kicks (Ch. 2)
- Seated Leg Lifts (Ch. 5)
- 3-Way Hip Kicks (Ch. 3)
- Mini Lunges (Ch.3)

Day 4

- Seated Leg Taps (Ch. 5)
- Narrow Stance Reach (Ch. 3)
- Lateral Stepping (Ch. 3)
- Heel Raises (Ch. 3)

Day 5

- Bridge (Ch. 5)
- Opposite Arm and Leg Raise (Ch. 5)
- Tandem Stance (Ch. 3)
- Walk on Tiptoes (Ch. 4)

BRAIN TRAINING WEEK

This week's schedule is focused on the brain and head movement. The exercises will include the vestibular moves that use the eyes and head in various manners as well as larger movements that include standing and walking exercises. Doing the eye and brain exercises first allows you to stop and recover from any dizziness before embarking on the larger movements required in the standing and walking ones.

Day 1
- Eyes Side-to-Side (Ch. 6)
- Eyes Up and Down (Ch. 6)
- Single Leg Stance (Ch. 3)
- Lateral Stepping (Ch. 3)

Day 2
- Gaze Stabilization Sitting (Ch. 6)
- Smooth Pursuits (Ch. 6)
- Trunk Circles (Ch. 2)
- Tandem Stance (Ch. 3)

Day 3
- Head and Eyes Same Direction (Ch. 6)
- Head and Eyes Opposite Direction (Ch. 6)
- Narrow Stance Reach (Ch. 3)
- Standing Marches (Ch. 3)

Day 4
- Head Bend (Ch. 6)
- Head Turn (Ch. 6)
- Mini Lunges (Ch. 3)
- Heel-to-Toe (Ch. 4)

Day 5
- Shoulder Turns (Ch. 6)
- Gaze Stabilization Standing (Ch. 6)
- Sit-to-Stand (Ch. 2)
- Foot Taps (Ch. 3)

WALKING AND MOVEMENT WEEK

Working on your balance while walking requires you to do several things at the same time. Before attempting this week's routine, be sure that you are at a comfortable level in your stability and are able to do all the seated, standing, core, and vestibular exercises.

Day 1

- Hip External Rotator Stretch (Ch. 2)
- Grapevine (Ch. 4)
- 3-Way Hip Kick (Ch. 3)
- Dynamic Walking (Ch. 4)

Day 2

- Squats (Ch. 3)
- Walk on Heels and Tiptoes (Ch. 4)
- Standing Marches (Ch. 3)
- Side Steps (Ch. 4)

Day 3

- Heel Raises (Ch. 3)
- Balance Walk (Ch. 4)
- Heel-to-Toe (Ch. 4)
- Ball Toss (Ch. 4)

Day 4

- Seated Forward Roll Ups (Ch. 5)
- Curb Walk (Ch. 4)
- Grapevine (Ch. 4)
- Backward Walking (Ch. 4)

Day 5

- Seated Side Bends (Ch. 5)
- Dynamic Walking (Ch. 4)
- Side Steps (Ch. 4)
- Zigzag Walk (Ch. 4)

Conclusion

We can't avoid age. However, we can avoid some aging. Continue to do things. Be active. Life is fantastic in the way it adjusts to demands; if you use your muscles and mind, they stay there much longer.

—Charles H. Townes

Well done, reader, on taking the initiative to regain and maintain your balance! By being your own advocate for healthy living and wellness maintenance, you have taken charge of your body and its well being. As we learned throughout the book, there are many things we can do to help our bodies remain strong and stable even as we get older. Aging doesn't have to mean fading, health-wise. Remaining active and engaging in regular physical activity can result in longevity, adding years to your life. Equally important, however, is that by continuing to exercise and be active, you are adding life to your remaining years.

We learned early on in the book that by keeping a regular exercise routine, we can accomplish things like:

- Helping prevent illness and disease
- Encouraging good mental health
- Improving cognitive functioning
- Lessening the risk of falling
- Staying connected with others

Older adults can hold many misconceptions about exercise, including thoughts of being too old or too weak. The reality is that exercise is what keeps us youthful in mind and spirit, helps ward off illness and chronic disease, and maintains our weight and balance in the long run. By including exercise in the key four areas of cardiovascular, strength training, flexibility, and balance, we can stay healthy and productive for the remainder of our lives. We learned that exercise doesn't have to be strenuous or hard to be effective, which is good news especially for those with medical problems or limited mobility. Any kind of movement is good for the body.

In learning about how our body regulates balance, we saw that there are many layers to everything in our body working together. The sensory information that we get from our eyes, ears, skin, muscles, and joints all get sent to the the brain, which then processes that input. After integrating all the bits and pieces of information, the brain sends messages to the rest of the body, including the arms, legs, feet, and core, as to what responses to make, or what things to adjust, to keep everything stable.

Next, we looked at the reality and consequences of falling because of the loss of balance. The data on the fall rates of those over 65 years old shows that a quarter of the older population falls every year and will continue to experience falls after the initial one. The consequences of falling can be serious injury to the brain, broken bones, internal bleeding, and potentially the loss of independence because of the fall outcome. Many factors contribute to the fall risk factors including: reduced or poor vision, foot problems, medication side-effects, vitamin D deficiency, and tripping hazards in the home. Preventative measures can be taken to reduce the likelihood of tripping and falling, such as getting an eye exam, checking with your doctor about your medications and vitamin D supplements, and making needed changes in your home to reduce the risk of falls.

The balance test at the end of Chapter 1 gave us an idea of how robust our balance was currently and the following chapters outlined how we can effectively boost our body's ability to remain stable while sitting, standing, and walking.

The balance exercises we learned in this book comprised of:

- Seated exercises. The 10 exercises in this chapter concentrated on simple movements to train and retrain our muscles for stability from a seated position.

- Standing exercises. Progressing to a standing position, we worked on specific exercises that mimic everyday activities and tasks while building balance on our feet.

- Walking exercises. These exercises incorporated movement in the standing position and had us moving in small and big ways as our body practiced it's balance while walking.

- Core exercises. Because our core muscles, those in our abdomen, back, and glutes, hold our body upright, we worked on strengthening our core in ways that are back- and neck-friendly.

- Vestibular exercises. The last type of exercises concentrated on our eyes, ears, and brain, also known as the vestibular system. A stable vestibular system is key to good balance and control.

Lastly, we talked about how to implement all that we have learned in this book into a daily program. Depending on your goals, you can choose to incorporate the exercises into your fitness routine in a variety of ways. Adding in one exercise a day is a simple way to get started and allows you to methodically work through each exercise until you complete all fifty. Another option was to implement the exercises on a chapter-by-chapter basis. For those looking for a plug and play program, we looked at a month's worth of balance exercise routines that outline a weekly and daily schedule of what to do.

My hope and desire is that you have benefitted not only from the information and encouragement in this book, but that you also make these exercises a part of your daily life in regaining and maintaining your balance.

Please consider leaving me a review! I'd love to hear what you thought of the book and how it has helped you.

Scan the QR code:

I hope you enjoy good health and happiness on the long road ahead of you, and I wish you all the best. Thank you for allowing me toshare my knowledge with you.

Baz Thompson

References

16 positive quotes about ageing. (2019, May 9). Brightwatergroup.com. https://brightwatergroup.com/news-articles/16-positive-quotes-about-ageing/

Akdeniz, S., Hepguler, S., Öztürk, C., & Atamaz, F. C. (2016). The relation between vitamin D and postural balance according to clinical tests and tetrax posturography. Journal of Physical Therapy Science, 28(4), 1272–1277. https://doi.org/10.1589/jpts.28.1272

Baker, J. (2020, October 19). Why you need to test your balance (plus 3 exercises to improve it). Whole Life Challenge. https://www.wholelifechallenge.com/why-you-need-to-test-your-balance-plus-3-exercises-to-improve-it/

Balance exercises for stroke patients: How to improve stability. (2020, June 3). Flint Rehab. https://www.flintrehab.com/balance-exercises-for-stroke-patients/

Balance tests: MedlinePlus lab test information. (2019). Medlineplus.gov. https://medlineplus.gov/lab-tests/balance-tests/

Bedosky, L. (2021, March 13). The best core exercises for seniors. Get Healthy U | Chris Freytag. https://gethealthyu.com/best-core-exercises-for-seniors/

Betty Friedan quotes. (n.d.). BrainyQuote. https://www.brainyquote.com/quotes/betty_friedan_383994?src=t_aging

Bumgardner, W. (2020, May 29). 10 fun ways to add balance exercises to your walks. Verywell Fit. https://www.verywellfit.com/add-balance-exercises-to-your-walks-4142274

CDC. (2019a). Important facts about falls. Cdc.gov. https://www.cdc.gov/homeandrecreationalsafety/falls/adultfalls.html

CDC. (2019b). Older adults: Physical activity and health. Surgeon General report. Centers for Disease Control and Prevention. https://www.cdc.gov/nccdphp/sgr/olderad.htm

Centers for Disease Control. (n.d.). What you can do to prevent falls. https://www.cdc.gov/steadi/pdf/STEADI-Brochure-WhatYouCanDo-508.pdf

Charles H. Townes quotes. (n.d.). BrainyQuote. Retrieved November 6, 2021, from https://www.brainyquote.com/quotes/charles_h_townes_639625?src=t_aging

Continued vestibular rehabilitation exercises -level 1 general information for eye exercises. (n.d.). https://ahc.aurorahealthcare.org/fywb/x20521.pdf

David Linley quotes. (n.d.). BrainyQuote. Retrieved November 6, 2021, from https://

www.brainyquote.com/quotes/david_linley_1145134

Eartha Kitt quotes. (n.d.). BrainyQuote. Retrieved November 6, 2021, from https://www.brainyquote.com/quotes/eartha_kitt_474182

Elsawy, B., & Higgins, K. E. (2010). Physical activity guidelines for older adults. American Family Physician, 81(1), 55–59. https://www.aafp.org/afp/2010/0101/p55.html

Fratacelli, T. (2019, May 19). 12 balance exercises for seniors | with printable pictures and PDF. PTProgress | Career Development, Education, Health. https://www.pt-progress.com/balance-exercises-for-seniors/

George Burns quotes. (n.d.). BrainyQuote. Retrieved November 6, 2021, from https://www.brainyquote.com/quotes/george_burns_103932?src=t_getting_older

Gottberg, K. (2016, November 4). 50 of the best positive aging quotes I could find. SMART Living 365. https://www.smartliving365.com/50-best-positive-aging-quotes-find/

Hoffman, H. (2017, July 18). 5 best sitting balance exercises for stroke patients (with videos) | saebo. Saebo. https://www.saebo.com/blog/5-best-sitting-balance-exercises-stroke-patients-videos/

Peter Diamandis quotes. (n.d.). BrainyQuote. Retrieved November 6, 2021, from https://www.brainyquote.com/quotes/peter_diamandis_690491

Robinson, L. (2019). Senior exercise and fitness tips. HelpGuide.org. https://www.helpguide.org/articles/healthy-living/exercise-and-fitness-as-you-age.htm

Schrift, D. (2019). 12 best elderly balance exercises for seniors to reduce the risk of falls. Eldergym® Senior Fitness. https://eldergym.com/elderly-balance/

The best core exercises for older adults. (2021, April 1). Harvard Health. https://www.health.harvard.edu/staying-healthy/the-best-core-exercises-for-older-adults

The GreenFields. (2016). 5 benefits of exercise for seniors and aging adults | the greenfields continuing care community | lancaster, NY. Thegreenfields.org. https://thegreenfields.org/5-benefits-exercise-seniors-aging-adults/

Vestibular_Exercises. (n.d.). University of Mississippi Medical Center. Retrieved October 27, 2021, from https://www.umc.edu/Healthcare/ENT/Patient-Handouts/Adult/Otology/Vestibular_Exercises.html

Villines, Z. (2020, October 20). Balance problems: Symptoms, diagnosis, and treatment. Www.medicalnewstoday.com. https://www.medicalnewstoday.com/articles/balance-problems#when-to-see-a-doctor

Watson, M. A., Black, F. O., & Crowson, M. (n.d.). The human balance system. VeDA.

https://vestibular.org/article/what-is-vestibular/the-human-balance-system/the-human-balance-system-how-do-we-maintain-our-balance/

3 Easy Quad Stretches to Improve Thigh Flexibility. (2018). Verywell Fit. https://www.verywellfit.com/quadricep-stretches-2696366

American Council on Exercise. (2014, October 7). Top 10 Benefits of Stretching. Www.acefitness.org. https://www.acefitness.org/education-and-resources/lifestyle/blog/5107/top-10-benefits-of-stretching/

American Heart Association. (2014). Warm Up, Cool Down. Www.heart.org. https://www.heart.org/en/healthy-living/fitness/fitness-basics/warm-up-cool-down

Axtell, B. (2017, July 11). Foot Exercises: Strengthening, Flexibility, and More. Healthline. https://www.healthline.com/health/fitness-exercise/foot-exercises#toe-raise-point-and-curl

Batista, L. H., Vilar, A. C., de Almeida Ferreira, J. J., Rebelatto, J. R., & Salvini, T. F. (2009). Active stretching improves flexibility, joint torque, and functional mobility in older women. American Journal of Physical Medicine & Rehabilitation, 88(10), 815–822. https://doi.org/10.1097/PHM.0b013e3181b72149

Bumgardner, W. (2007, July 23). Shin Stretches for Your Anterior Tibialis. Verywell Fit; Verywell Fit. https://www.verywellfit.com/shin-stretches-standing-stetch-3436425

Cobra Abdominal Stretch / Old Horse Stretch – WorkoutLabs Exercise Guide. (n.d.). WorkoutLabs. Retrieved July 12, 2021, from https://workoutlabs.com/exercise-guide/cobra-abdominal-stretch/

Cronkleton, E. (2018, November 21). How to Get Rid of Lactic Acid in the Muscles. Healthline. https://www.healthline.com/health/how-to-get-rid-of-lactic-acid#warm-up

Cronkleton, E. (2019, July 12). Warmup Exercises: 6 Ways to Get Warmed Up Before a Workout. Healthline. https://www.healthline.com/health/fitness-exercise/warm-up-exercises#benefits

Davidson, K. (2021, April 20). Superman Exercise: How to Do It, Benefits, and Muscles Worked. Healthline. https://www.healthline.com/health/fitness/superman-exercise#muscles-worked

Eske, J. (2018, November 15). Best stretches for tight hamstrings: 7 methods. Www.medicalnewstoday.com. https://www.medicalnewstoday.com/articles/323703#7-best-hamstring-stretches

Evans, R. (2014, August 19). 4 Upper Back Stretches You Can Do at Your Desk. Healthline. https://www.healthline.com/health/back-pain/deskercize-upper-back#butterfly-wings

Gordon, D. (2021, January 28). 5 Ways to Perform Chest Stretches - wikiHow Fitness. Www.wikihow.fitness. https://www.wikihow.fitness/Perform-Chest-Stretches

Gudmestad, J. (2008, March 11). How to Stay Safe in Neck Rolls + Stretches | Yoga for your Neck. Yoga Journal. https://www.yogajournal.com/teach/how-to-stay-safe-in-neck-rolls-stretches/

Half Kneeling Hip Flexor Stretch | Functional Movement Systems. (n.d.). Www.functionalmovement.com. Retrieved July 7, 2021, from https://www.functionalmovement.com/Exercises/788/half_kneeling_hip_flexor_stretch

Harvard Health Publishing. (2013, September). The importance of stretching - Harvard Health. Harvard Health; Harvard Health. https://www.health.harvard.edu/staying-healthy/the-importance-of-stretching

Harvard Health Publishing. (2020, April 20). 5 exercises to improve hand mobility. Harvard Health. https://www.health.harvard.edu/pain/5-exercises-to-improve-hand-mobility

Higuera, V. (2020, November 23). Happy Baby Pose: How to Do, Benefits, and History. Healthline. https://www.healthline.com/health/happy-baby-pose

Hip Rotations. (n.d.). Www.workoutaholic.net. Retrieved July 13, 2021, from https://www.workoutaholic.net/exercises/hip_rotations

How to do Seated Spinal Twist. (n.d.). ClassPass. https://classpass.com/movements/seated-spinal-twist

How to do Thread the Needle Pose. (n.d.). ClassPass. Retrieved July 8, 2021, from https://classpass.com/movements/thread-the-needle-pose

Inverarity, L. (2005, November 23). Iliotibial (IT) Band Stretches to Treat ITBS. Verywell Fit; Verywell Fit. https://www.verywellfit.com/iliotibial-band-stretches-2696360

Lee, S. B., Oh, J. H., Park, J. H., Choi, S. P., & Wee, J. H. (2018). Differences in youngest-old, middle-old, and oldest-old patients who visit the emergency department. Clinical and Experimental Emergency Medicine, 5(4), 249–255. https://doi.org/10.15441/ceem.17.261

LoElizabeth. (2016, August 24). How To Yoga Fundamentals: Reclined Figure-4 To Prevent Injury. LoElizabeth Blog. http://loelizabeth.com/figure-4/

Lower Body Stretches. (n.d.). Www.arthritis.org. https://www.arthritis.org/health-wellness/healthy-living/physical-activity/success-strategies/lower-body-stretches

Marturana, A. (2019). 10 Great Stretches to Do After an Upper-Body Workout. SELF. https://www.self.com/gallery/upper-body-stretches

McCormick, R., & Vasilaki, A. (2018). Age-related changes in skeletal muscle: changes to life-style as a therapy. Biogerontology, 19(6), 519–536. https://doi.org/10.1007/s10522-018-9775-3

Meyler, Z. (2018, September 14). 4 Easy Stretches for a Stiff Neck. Spine-Health. https://www.spine-health.com/wellness/exercise/4-easy-stretches-stiff-neck

Miller, R. (2020, June 5). Easy Hamstring Stretches. Spine-Health. https://www.spine-health.com/wellness/exercise/easy-hamstring-stretches

National Center for Biotechnology Information, U.S. National Library of Medicine. (2020). What happens when you age? In www.ncbi.nlm.nih.gov. Institute for Quality and Efficiency in Health Care (IQWiG). https://www.ncbi.nlm.nih.gov/books/NBK563107/

Overhead Stretch. (n.d.). Www.exercise.com. https://www.exercise.com/exercises/overhead-stretch/

Pizer, A. (2021, May 24). How to Do Paschimottanasana, a Yoga Hamstring Stretch. Verywell Fit. https://www.verywellfit.com/seated-forward-bend-paschimottanasana-3567101

Posture of the Month: Banana Pose. (2018, October 5). Your Pace Yoga. https://yourpaceyoga.com/blog/posture-of-the-month-banana-pose/

Quinn, E. (2019a). The Basic Bridge Exercise for Core Stability. Verywell Fit. https://www.verywellfit.com/how-to-do-the-bridge-exercise-3120738

Quinn, E. (2019b, August 31). How to Do the Standing Lunge Stretch. Verywell Fit. https://www.verywellfit.com/performing-standing-lunge-stretch-3120306

Raye, J. (n.d.). Yin Yoga Square Pose with modifications. Jennifer Raye | Medicine and Movement. Retrieved July 12, 2021, from https://jenniferraye.com/blog/square-pose

Reclined Butterfly Pose. (n.d.). Ekhart Yoga. Retrieved July 8, 2021, from https://www.ekhartyoga.com/resources/yoga-poses/reclined-butterfly-pose

Schwengel, K. (2017, August 28). Lymph Flow Exercise: Floor Angels | Natural Balance Therapy. Naturalbalancetherapy.com. https://naturalbalancetherapy.com/self-treatment/lymph-flow-exercise-floor-angels/

Sleep Advisor. (2020, June 3). 8 Stretches for Your Best Night's Sleep. Sleep Advisor. https://www.sleepadvisor.org/stretching-before-bed/

Standing Twists / Trunk Rotations (Barbell) | Chunk Fitness. (2021). Chunkfitness.com. https://chunkfitness.com/exercises/ab-exercises/oblique-exercises/standing-twists-trunk-rotations-barbell

Stretch of the Week: Windshield Wiper Stretch. (2016, April 13). Athletico. https://

www.athletico.com/2016/04/13/stretch-week-windshield-wiper-stretch/

Stretch22. (n.d.). The Top Benefits of Stretching in the Morning. Stretch 22. Retrieved July 7, 2021, from https://stretch22.com/wake-and-stretch-the-top-benefits-of-stretching-in-the-morning/

Sugar, J. (2018, December 23). This Is Our Favorite Stretch to Do in Bed: Cat and Cow. POPSUGAR Fitness. https://www.popsugar.com/fitness/Relieve-Back-Pain-Cat-Cow-Stretch-8320711

Supine Spinal Twist Can Help Improve Back Mobility. (n.d.). Verywell Fit. Retrieved July 8, 2021, from https://www.verywellfit.com/supine-spinal-twist-supta-matsyendrasana-3567125

Tight Shoulders: 12 Stretches for Fast Relief and Tips for Prevention. (2018, January 12). Healthline. https://www.healthline.com/health/tight-shoulders#stretches

Top 10 shoulder stretches for pain and tightness. (2019, March 8). Www.medicalnewstoday.com. https://www.medicalnewstoday.com/articles/324647#shoulder-rolls

Tucker, A. (2018). 5 Essential Calf Stretches Everyone Should Be Doing. SELF. https://www.self.com/gallery/essential-calf-stretches

Volpi, E., Nazemi, R., & Fujita, S. (2004). Muscle tissue changes with aging. Current Opinion in Clinical Nutrition and Metabolic Care, 7(4), 405–410. https://doi.org/10.1097/01.mco.0000134362.76653.b2

Walker, B. (2010, August 27). What is stretching? How to stretch properly? When to stretch? Stretch Coach. https://stretchcoach.com/articles/how-to-stretch/

Yoga Poses Dictionary | Pocket Yoga. (n.d.). Www.pocketyoga.com. Retrieved July 6, 2021, from https://www.pocketyoga.com/pose/mountain_cactus_arms

5 Core Exercises for Seniors: Build Strength From Your Center. (n.d.). Retrieved February 19, 2022, from Snug Safety website: http://www.snugsafe.com/all-posts/core-exercises-for-seniors

6 Core Stretches That Will Make Your Abs Feel Amazing. (n.d.). Retrieved February 19, 2022, from LIVESTRONG.COM website: http://www.livestrong.com/article/355186-core-muscle-stretches

Arana, J. (2020, June 25). How to Tone Abs While Walking. Retrieved February 19, 2022, from wikiHow website: http://www.wikihow.com/Tone-Abs-While-Walking

Back Exercises: Neck and Torso Rotation. (n.d.). Retrieved February 19, 2022, from demo.staywellhealthlibrary.com website: https://demo.staywellhealthlibrary.com/Content/healthsheets-v1/neck-exercises-necktorso-rotation/

Barroa_Artworks. (2022). Retrieved February 15, 2022, from Pixabay.com website: https://cdn.pixabay.com/photo/2018/01/31/07/53/muscle-3120521_960_720.png

Bedosky, L. (2021, March 13). The Best Core Exercises for Seniors. Retrieved from Get Healthy U | Chris Freytag website: https://gethealthyu.com/best-core-exercises-for-seniors/

Bubnis, D. (2016, February 11). 29 Full-Body Partner Exercises. Retrieved February 19, 2022, from Greatist website: https://greatist.com/fitness/35-kick-ass-partner-exercises

Bubnis, D. (2020, April 11). When's the Best Time to Exercise? Retrieved February 13, 2022, from Greatist website: https://greatist.com/fitness/whats-best-time-work-out

Capritto, A. (2020, November 24). 4 important benefits of a strong core. Retrieved February 13, 2022, from CNET website: https://www.cnet.com/health/fitness/why-you-really-need-a-strong-core-for-fitness-and-life/

Davis, N. (2020, October 23). Try This: 24 Standing Ab Exercises to Strengthen and Define Your Core. Retrieved February 19, 2022, from Healthline website: https://www.healthline.com/health/fitness-exercise/standing-ab-exercises#stretch.

Dilthey, M. R. (2020, January 23). Is It Better to Do Your Ab Workout in the Morning or at Night? Retrieved from LIVESTRONG.COM website: https://www.livestrong.com/article/301734-the-best-time-to-work-out-abs/

Exercise Library:Cobra. (n.d.). Retrieved from www.acefitness.org website: https://www.acefitness.org/education-and-resources/lifestyle/exercise-library/16/cobra/

Exercise Library:Leg Crossover Stretch. (n.d.). Retrieved February 10, 2022, from www.acefitness.org website: https://www.acefitness.org/education-and-resources/lifestyle/exercise-library/231/leg-crossover-stretch/

Ferraro, K. (2021, September 11). The 10 Benefits of a Strong Core, According to Trainers. Retrieved from Byrdie website: https://www.byrdie.com/benefits-of-a-strong-core-5189502

Fetters, A. (2017, September 25). The 10-Minute Seated Core Workout. Retrieved February 19, 2022, from SilverSneakers website: http://www.silversneakers.com/blog/10-minute-chair-core-workout

Fetters, A. (2019, March 12). 6 Core Exercises to Ease Lower Back Pain. Retrieved February 19, 2022, from SilverSneakers website: http://www.silversneakers.com/blog/core-exercises-ease-back-pain

Harvard Health, P. (2012, January 12). The real-world benefits of strengthening your core. Retrieved from Harvard Health website: https://www.health.harvard.edu/healthbeat/the-real-world-benefits-of-strengthening-your-core

Kissam, B. (2018, September 17). 0-6 Pack Abs Phase 1 - Miracle Muscles | Warrior Made. Retrieved February 19, 2022, from results.warriormade.com website: https://results.warriormade.com/0-6pack-abs/phase1-miracle-muscles/

Lefkowith, C. (2015, July 22). 20 Partner Exercises | Redefining Strength. Retrieved from Redefining Strength website: https://redefiningstrength.com/try-these-20-partner-exercises-for-a-fun-full-body-workout/

Malacoff, J. (2018, April 24). 6 Signs You Need to Strengthen Your Core | Fitness | MyFitnessPal. Retrieved from MyFitnessPal Blog website: https://blog.myfitnesspal.com/6-signs-you-need-to-strengthen-your-core/

Maurice. (2021, February 1). Core Exercises for Seniors: Complete Guide to Ab Exercises for Seniors -. Retrieved from Seniors Mobility website: https://seniorsmobility.org/exercises/core-exercises-for-seniors/

McCormick, R., & Vasilaki, A. (2018). Age-related changes in skeletal muscle: changes to life-style as a therapy. Biogerontology, 19(6), 519–536. https://doi.org/10.1007/s10522-018-9775-3

Miller, B. (2016, January 29). 6 Ways To Tone Your Abs While You Walk. Retrieved from Prevention website: https://www.prevention.com/fitness/a20496857/tone-your-abs-while-walking/

Moreland, B., Kakara, R., & Henry, A. (2020). Trends in Nonfatal Falls and Fall-Related Injuries Among Adults Aged ≥65 Years — United States, 2012–2018. MMWR. Morbidity and Mortality Weekly Report, 69(27), 875–881. https://doi.org/10.15585/mmwr.mm6927a5

Nunez, K. (2021, September 27). Best Core Exercises: Top Moves, from Beginner to Advanced. Retrieved February 19, 2022, from Healthline website: https://www.healthline.com/health/best-core-exercises#Bicycle-crunch.

Partner Workout with Kelli & Daniel - Fitness Blender's 100th Free Full Length Workout Video. (2012, July 9). Retrieved February 19, 2022, from www.youtube.com website: http://www.youtube.com/watch?v=tD-4Vm0AY28

Pizer, A. (2020, March 27). The Child's Pose for Resting in Yoga. Retrieved from Verywell Fit website: https://www.verywellfit.com/childs-pose-balasana-3567066

Pizer, A. (2021, December 8). How to Do Cat-Cow Stretch (Chakravakasana) in Yoga. Retrieved from Verywell Fit website: https://www.verywellfit.com/cat-cow-stretch-chakravakasana-3567178

Search Results. (n.d.). Retrieved February 12, 2022, from BrainyQuote website:

https://www.brainyquote.com/search_results?x=0&y=0&q=aging+strong

Slide show: Exercises to improve your core strength. (2020, August 11). Retrieved from Mayo Clinic website: https://www.mayoclinic.org/healthy-lifestyle/fitness/multimedia/core-strength/sls-20076575?s=8

The best core exercises for older adults. (2021, April 1). Retrieved from Harvard Health website: https://www.health.harvard.edu/staying-healthy/the-best-core-exercises-for-older-adults

Townsend, H. (2020, June 16). 7 Standing Core Exercises for Seniors. Retrieved February 19, 2022, from SilverSneakers website: https://www.silversneakers.com/blog/7-standing-exercises-for-core-strength

www.ingramcontent.com/pod-product-compliance
Lightning Source LLC
Chambersburg PA
CBHW080416030426
42335CB00020B/2476